Second Edition

Sports Conditioning and Weight Training

PROGRAMS FOR ATHLETIC COMPETITION

WILLIAM J. STONE

Department of Health, Physical Education
Arizona State University

Consultant—
Phoenix SUNS, NBA
Sportsmedicine Clinic, Phoenix

WILLIAM A. KROLL

Strength Coach
University of Illinois

59   176

Allyn and Bacon, Inc.   Boston   London   Sydney   Toronto

Photographs for the second edition were taken by John C. Dixon.

Copyright © 1986 by Allyn and Bacon, Inc.,
7 Wells Avenue, Newton, Massachusetts 02159

Library of Congress Cataloging in Publication Data

Stone, William J., 1937–
  Sports conditioning and weight training.

  Bibliography: p.
  1. Physical education and training.   2. Exercise.
3. Weight lifting.   I. Kroll, William A., 1944–
II. Title.
GV711.5.S76   1986   613.7'1   85-13430
ISBN 0-205-08424-9

Printed in the United States of America

10 9 8 7 6 5 4 3 2   90 89 88 87 86

Contents

Preface

Since the publication of the first edition, there has been a veritable explosion of interest in the field of sports conditioning. There has developed a national association for strength and conditioning, which now publishes the *National Strength & Conditioning Association Journal.* Other publications have developed as outlets for research and communication concerning sports conditioning. The number of conditioning equipment manufacturers continues to proliferate.

The authors are gratified to note that many of the concepts proposed in the first edition are currently endorsed by conditioning experts. The authors also think that the second edition is a significant improvement over the first. What began as a standard revision became a major overhaul as a result of an avalanche of new information flooding the field.

In addition to bringing the material in each of the original chapters up-to-date, the authors have added several new features. New chapters included in Part I are: Chapter 5: Flexibility, Warm-Up, and Stretching and Chapter 7: Sports Nutrition. Chapter 10: Soccer has been added to Part II. Sections on de-conditioning and overtraining have been added to Chapter 8: The Conditioning Program, which deals with year-round training. For those who seek additional information and expertise in specific sports, sport-specific references have been added to the program chapters (Chapters 9–17). In response to both current needs and reader requests, it is anticipated that this second edition will better serve the needs of the athlete or coach.

This book is designed to offer sound, systematic training programs for those who wish to *apply* strength and conditioning techniques to *specific* sports. It should be, by design, a practical volume for the coach or athlete who wishes to use it in his or her sport. The programs offered in this volume are *basic* and simple, in order to meet the needs of *men* and *women* athletes in a wide age range.

The widespread use of supplementary training of men for sports is not of recent origin. Female athletes and coaches, however, are, for the most part, relative newcomers to highly competitive athletic programs and intense training regimens. Many athletes and coaches of both sexes are influenced by the training regimens of high-level performers in their sport. The major considerations in the adoption of a training program are whether the program is scientifically sound, and whether it is appropriate to the age and sex of the athlete or team. The authors have made a major effort to describe the scientific bases of sports conditioning in readable fashion and then to outline easily followed conditioning programs for specific sports.

Part I of this volume is designed to furnish the scientific foundations of conditioning and strength building. It outlines the rationale for supplementary training for athletes and describes the exercises and techniques used in Part II. The programs described in Part II are geared to specific sports and can easily be used by the novice with guidance from Part I. Those athletes with no prior weight training experience are cautioned to seek help from coaches or experienced weight trainers before attempting unfamiliar weight exercises. Athletes should not use high intensity conditioning programs if they have cardiorespiratory problems that limit their physical activity.

The authors are very cognizant of the need for a practical source for conditioning men and women. They have studied extensively the theoretical bases of conditioning and have tested the techniques offered here under practical conditions. Perhaps of more importance to many readers, they also combine many years of experience in the conditioning of topflight professional, college, and high school athletes. They envision that the book will be a valuable aid to coaches and athletes who strive for excellence in their sport.

William J. Stone
William A. Kroll

PART

I

FOUNDATIONS OF CONDITIONING AND STRENGTH BUILDING

Chapter 1 deals with the rationale for supplementary training for sports and the scientific bases of conditioning and strength building. The second chapter describes the structure and content of the muscles and cardiorespiratory systems, and what happens to those systems as a result of training. In Chapters 3 and 4 attention is drawn to the basic techniques of conditioning and strength development. In the fifth chapter the distinction is drawn between flexibility, warm-up, and stretching. Injury prevention and rehabilitation techniques are discussed in Chapter 6. The final chapter in this section deals with sports nutrition and explores a number of questions frequently asked by coaches and athletes.

1

Sports Conditioning

This book is written for YOU, the athlete or coach. Part I is designed to aid you in using the conditioning programs listed in Part II. The background information is intended to give you a basic understanding of the scientific principles involved in training. The specific techniques should enable the novice to initiate a conditioning program that is scientifically sound and easy to follow. This chapter will discuss the need for physical conditioning in sports and will define some of the basic goals of sports conditioning.

SPORTS CONDITIONING: THE RATIONALE

The past several decades have shown a vast improvement in sports performances, and numerous records have been set. While that statement could be made at any point in the history of sport, there has been a noticeable acceleration in the rate at which records have been broken. Those sports in which records are kept and can be compared include primarily track and field and swimming.

Recorded performances improve over time for many reasons, such as bigger athletes, better nutrition, improved coaching techniques, and more scientific conditioning programs. It is frequently pointed out that men's gold medal winners of past Olympic swimming events would be hard pressed to place in a respectable position in current Olympic Games, in the women's division! Obviously training and conditioning programs have played a major role in the improved performances in sport. It is impractical to compare teams and athletes in many other sports with their counterparts from the past, but the indications are that their increased

size, speed, power, and conditioning have resulted in superior performances.[7]

Much of the impetus for improved conditioning techniques and better performance emerged from the decade of the 1950s. During that time interval training was being introduced into this country on a widespread basis; Roger Bannister broke the four-minute mile barrier in England; and a number of other performance barriers were cracked. Bannister's accomplishment came as a result of a careful and scientific approach to conditioning on the part of a pre-med student with a great deal of knowledge about exercise physiology. Strength training began to become a part of the preparation and conditioning of a number of outstanding amateur and professional athletes.

It may be difficult for younger athletes and coaches to imagine the earlier resistance to some of the techniques that are now commonplace in sports conditioning. Strength training was shunned by many athletes and coaches three decades ago. Today most professional and many college teams have a strength and/or conditioning coach. Scientific conditioning programs have become a standard practice from high school athletes to professionals. For most athletes and coaches, the conditioning results alone justify the time spent in sports conditioning. Sports scientists require a more stringent order of proof, and a significant amount of research data supports many of the current conditioning approaches.[11] Some practices are less well documented and will require additional investigation before sports scientists are satisfied that they are effective. The authors take the position that sports conditioning promoters cannot take sole credit for improved performance but that a scientifically devised program can contribute to performance.

A major objective in this text is to review the scientific bases of conditioning and their application to sports conditioning programs.

Perhaps one of the most dramatic examples of the importance of conditioning in sport occurred during the 1970s. For many years the Soviet ice hockey team had made regular visits to the United States to challenge college hockey teams. The Soviets were almost always victorious. When a series of games with "Team Canada" was started in the 1970s, the Soviets were given little chance to win against the National Hockey League professionals who made up the Canadian group. The first series proved to be eye-opening for United States and Canadian hockey observers. The highly disciplined Soviets, skating relentlessly, were able to win several games primarily on the basis of superior physical conditioning. Games that were close in the first period became a rout in the third period as the better-conditioned Soviets outskated the NHL professionals.

SPORTS VS. CONDITIONING REQUIREMENTS OF SPORT

It has long been recognized that actual practice of a sport is the best means of preparing for the skills and strategies needed for the game. Some sports, however, do not make sufficient demands upon all of the physiological systems supporting the performance. Thus there is the need to spend time in developing top physical condition. Conditioning exercises are necessary to increase the capacity of the supporting systems and, in many cases, the muscles directly involved.[9]

The amount of time spent in practice in order to develop skills and strategy versus physical conditioning will vary according to the physical demands of the sport. Runners and swimmers are constantly practicing their skills as they work out, but their performance will be determined primarily by their physical condition. Volleyball and basketball players probably do not require the high degree of physical conditioning needed by swimmers and runners, but conditioning is still an important component of their game. On the other side of the continuum from the highly physical sports are activities that require a great deal of attention to skills development (golf) but less concern for physical conditioning. (See Figure 1.1.) This spectrum of sports is best viewed as a continuum with both skills-strategy development and physical conditioning as basic preparation for all sports.

Hence, the baseball player strengthens his arms, wrists, and shoulders by performing weight training exercises rather than relying on the weight of the bat alone to furnish increased strength. The pitcher runs in order to increase his general endurance as well as the local muscular endurance in his

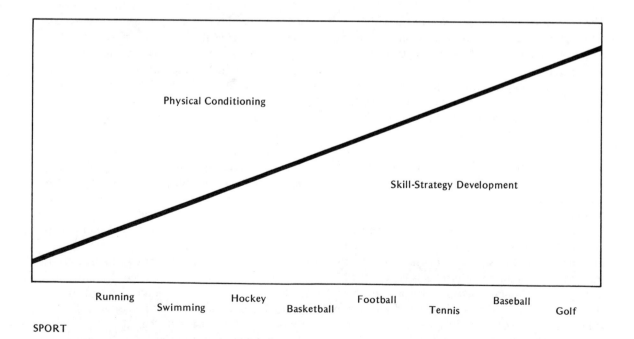

FIGURE 1.1 *Skill vs. Conditioning Requirements of Sports*

legs, knowing that there may be only limited opportunity for him to run during a game. Both of these conditioning factors are necessary for the baseball player but skills practice alone will usually not develop them sufficiently. The same rationale applies to a wide range of sports, including many that are far more vigorous than baseball. The platoon system in football reduces the amount of time actually spent in the game, yet the player on either offense or defense must be prepared for rigorous physical activity. The football player requires considerable endurance despite the fact that the ball is in play for only a few seconds at a time.

Although the use of weight training and physical conditioning programs has become very widespread in athletics, it should also be noted that practice does not automatically ensure better performance. The key element in making supplementary training a valuable contribution to the total program of preparing the athlete for competition is *specificity of training*.

Specificity in Athletic Performance and Conditioning

The most dominant characteristic of sports skills performance is a high degree of specificity. *Specificity* means that sports skills are highly unique; that no matter how much "alike" they appear, there are usually a number of minor differences that make it difficult to perform many skills well without a great deal of practice. Furthermore, one cannot carry over athletic performance from one sport to another unless the two are nearly identical.[2]

The concept of specificity is sometimes difficult to comprehend because of a number of multiskilled individuals who tend to excel in several sports. There is considerable evidence that such rare individuals are probably blessed with many specific skills and have practiced those skills a great deal. They are also highly motivated.

The staggering number of physical factors, such as arm speed, leg power, reaction time, and balance, that might be involved in various combinations in a single sports skill makes specificity quite logical. The fact that many psychological factors also play a role in athletic performance adds to the uniqueness of each sports skill and performance. The astute coach or athlete pays heed to the specificity of sports skills development by concentrating primarily on the actual practice of the sport. It should not be surprising that the same

principle must be applied to sports conditioning. Specificity in training refers, then, to matching the conditioning or strength demands of the sport to the training techniques.

Physical conditioning for any sport should match the physiological demands of the activity. Basketball, for example, requires a high level of general endurance but also includes brief periods of all-out activity such as occur during a fast break. Football, on the other hand, represents a series of all-out bursts of energy followed by brief recovery period. Recent work in muscle physiology lends support not only to sports conditioning but to specificity when preparing for sports performance. Research on muscle fiber typing indicates that endurance training affects one muscle fiber type while all-out training affects another fiber type.[4] This suggests strongly that if both qualities are needed in a sport, training must be designed for both. (Fiber typing is discussed in more detail in Chapter 2.) Of even greater concern to coaches and athletes is evidence that training systems are not complementary and may even be detrimental to the other training quality. Thus it becomes extremely important for the coach or athlete to weigh the amount of general endurance versus all-out power required in the sport. This factor is discussed in detail in Part II, wherein training programs are designed relative to the physical demands of each sport.

DEFINITIONS

A few descriptive definitions are in order here to prepare the reader for terms that will be used frequently throughout the book. The terms are briefly defined, synonymous terms are used, and brief explanations are given of their importance to athletic performance.

Aerobic Power

Aerobic power is the ability to maintain high work loads continuously for prolonged periods of time without becoming unduly fatigued. In sports terminology, this refers to the ability of an athlete to operate at high levels of activity during the game and to continue "putting out" without becoming prematurely "winded." Most team sports require a good-to-excellent aerobic capacity on the part of the athlete. Aerobic capacity is literally the basis

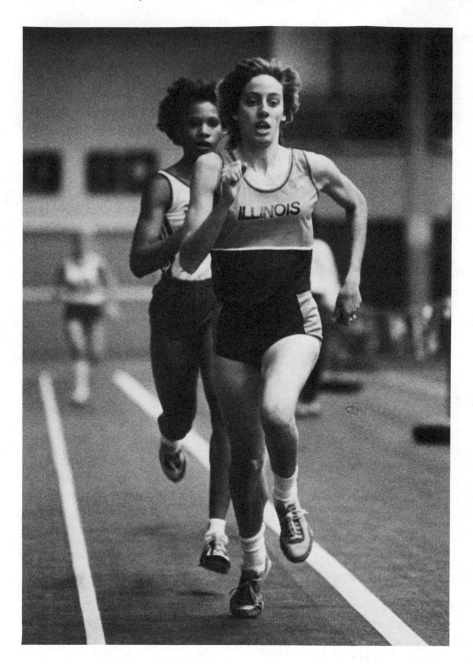

PHOTO 1.1   *Aerobic Power*

of good athletic performance, as most sports require moving the body almost continuously.

Sports medicine experts and exercise physiologists recognize aerobic power as the major index of general endurance or physical fitness. Aerobic capacity depends upon the ability of the heart and lungs to supply oxygen to the working muscles and is developed usually by large muscle, whole body movements like running, swimming, and cycling.

Anaerobic Power

Anaerobic power is the ability to work in excess of the body's capacity to take oxygen into the tissues, resulting in an oxygen debt. This type of work in sports is characterized by the performer going all out for brief periods of time, such as in a series of fast breaks in basketball. The capacity to operate anaerobically is limited to brief periods even in the most highly trained athlete. Anaerobic training can

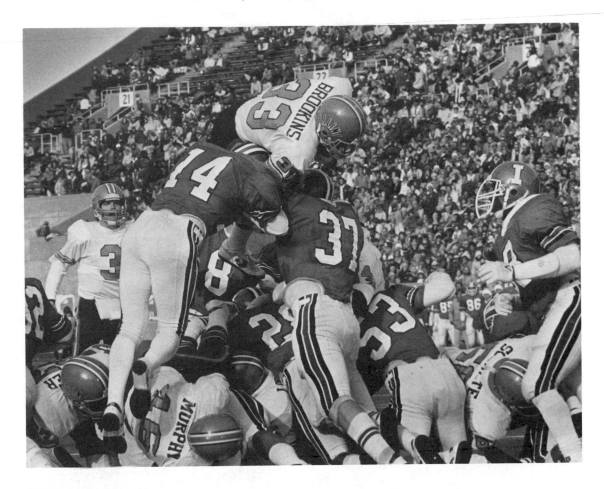

PHOTO 1.2 *Anaerobic Power*

increase the athlete's capacity to operate at intense levels and the training effect is brought about from physiological and psychological factors. The latter factor is an important one, since it involves a willingness to withstand the discomfort of going all out repeatedly.

If aerobic capacity is the basis of most performances, anaerobic capacity can be considered the frosting on the cake. At the highest levels of athletic competition, where the range of skill is narrow, willingness to tolerate anaerobic effort may provide the margin necessary to win or succeed.

Muscular Strength

Strength or *1 RM* refers to the maximum amount of tension the muscle or muscle group can apply in a single effort. Strength can be subdivided into two components: 1) *static strength*, meaning the maximum amount of tension the muscle can apply against resistance, involving little or no movement in the muscle, and 2) *dynamic strength*, referring to the application of great force through a full range of motion. Nearly all applications of strength in athletics are of this type. The athlete applies force through nearly a full range of motion and very rapidly, as is evident in throwing, jumping, running, kicking, and striking.

One of the major factors that distinguishes the skilled performer from the less skilled one is strength. It has been clearly established in a number of studies that strength training has a beneficial effect on motor skills and sports performance.[1] While it should not be inferred that strength is the cause of skill, the relationship held through all the age groups studied. Increased strength could be a prerequisite to better athletic performance. The same might be said of aerobic capacity. Better performance cannot be expected unless the athlete has sufficient strength and aerobic power to maintain lengthy practice sessions or game situations without undue fatigue. Strength training is anaerobic in nature and it affects the same fibers as anaerobic training.

Muscular Endurance

Muscular endurance refers to the capacity to continue submaximal muscle contractions repeatedly. It is associated with local areas of the body, such as the legs in running, swimming, or bicycling. Most athletic events require local muscular endurance in one or more areas of the body, and this endurance is developed by weight training or aerobic training. Although muscular endurance is on the opposite end of the continuum from strength, it can be greatly influenced by the strength of the local muscle group. If two athletes are applying force against the same resistance repeatedly, then the stronger of the two should fatigue less because he will be using a smaller percentage of his maximal strength with each effort. Muscular endurance is an important facet of athletic performance simply because actions are repeated over and over in a game.

Power

Power refers to work (force X distance) per unit of time. This is the application of great force in a very brief time span. In athletics, *explosive strength* is often used synonymously with the term *power*. The football lineman, basketball rebounder, and shot-putter come to mind most readily when describing explosive strength or power.

There is perhaps no other cluster of performances in athletics wherein strength building has greater potential to contribute toward better performance than those events requiring explosive strength. The great increase in dynamic strength that accrues from weight training can be utilized directly when applying force rapidly. Some of the earliest efforts to use supplementary weight training were designed to increase athletic power.

Speed

Speed refers to the rapidity with which one contracts a muscle or group of muscles. Running speed in sports is thus a series of rapid muscle contrac-

PHOTO 1.3   *Power/Explosive Strength*

tions. The time that it takes the athlete to move from one place to another is a measure of his or her speed, but there is another component of movement time, and that is *acceleration*.

Acceleration

Acceleration refers to increasing the velocity (speed), such as the sprinter leaving the starting blocks or the golf club accelerating as it approaches the ball. These same examples also involve explosive strength, which points out the interrelationship of strength-speed-power.

The importance of speed and acceleration in athletics is obvious, whether they involve the

PHOTO 1.4 *Speed*

PHOTO 1.5 *Acceleration*

athlete moving his body quickly or accelerating light objects such as rackets, clubs, bats, and balls. The strength-speed relationship is not nearly as clear, however, as that of strength and power. The relationship between strength and speed of limb movement is not particularly high when there is little resistance. With greater resistance, the contribution of strength to speed becomes greater. Thus the contribution of additional strength to limb speed may be greater for the shot-putter than for the baseball pitcher. The pitcher may still benefit, although gains in speed may not be proportional to gains in strength. The same principles may be said to apply to running speed. Since acceleration is a major factor in running short distances, the increased strength derived from training may be of

greater importance when overcoming inertia than at later stages when top running speed has been attained.

Flexibility

Flexibility refers to the range of motion in a joint or series of joints. Most athletic events require a dynamic range of motion. Flexibility can also be measured in the static mode by having the athlete reach slowly through a full range of motion. The importance of flexibility is very evident in those sports events that are judged aesthetically, such as gymnastics, diving, and figure skating. Flexibility

PHOTO 1.6   *Flexibility*

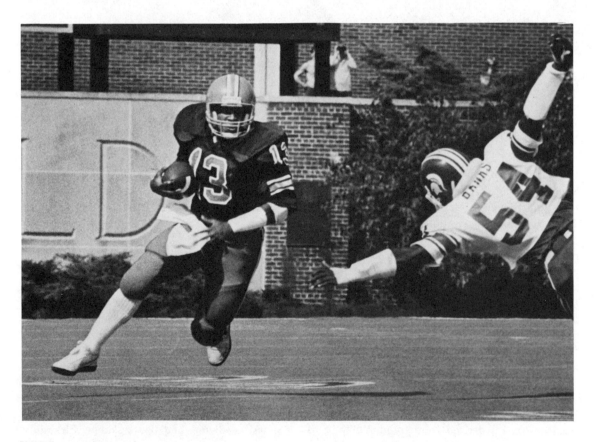

PHOTO 1.7   *Agility*

is also important in the majority of sports that value performance strictly on effect rather than form.

Agility

Agility involves rapid change of body direction or limb position. Greater acceleration of the body and greater speed of limb movement contribute to increased agility. The interrelationships of factors in sport performance should be evident. Control of the body can be dependent upon the strength of the supporting muscles in the arms, legs, or trunk. Most sports require a great deal of agility, for example, volleyball, basketball, baseball, football, and tennis.

THE DIMENSIONS OF ATHLETIC PERFORMANCE

Many factors contribute to athletic performance, some of which are defined above. It is not surprising then that there is as much specificity to both athletic performance and conditioning as there is, given the variety of ways those factors can contribute to different sport skills. In Figure 1.2 the authors have reduced a variety of factors into three dimensions: physical endowment, specific skill, and psychological endowment.

Figure 1.2 is intended to illustrate the importance of practicing the specific sports skill for improvement in athletic performance. The other dimensions are also important in determining the quality of the athletic performance. Physical endowment is highly important in athletic performance and many physical endowment factors can be improved by sports conditioning. While the athlete may not be able to influence height or body type, he or she can increase strength, speed, aerobic power, anaerobic power, and flexibility, among other factors. Those factors influence not only athletic performance in general but also specific sports skills. Psychological endowment, while also very important in athletic performance, is considerably more difficult for the coach, in particular, to influence. There is greater variability among athletes in behavioral response to athletic experiences than in physical conditioning.

In preparing for a sport, it is evident that the coach or athlete must be concerned with all three dimensions which contribute to athletic performance. It is fair to state that most of the time spent in preparation for sport goes into the development of skills and strategics. This is as it should be because that is what sports are all about. One of the objectives of this text is to encourage athletes and coaches to give more careful consideration to the physical dimension through sports conditioning.

FIGURE 1.2 *The Dimensions of Athletic Performance*

SPORTS CONDITIONING

The authors identify the major areas of sports conditioning as: aerobic power, anaerobic power, flexibility, and strength. See Figure 1.3. Many factors that are targeted for sports conditioning can be included in those four major headings. Anaerobic power can also include the development of speed, power, and acceleration. Aerobic power as well as strength will influence muscular endurance. Nearly every sport requires some level of conditioning in each of those four areas, although the emphasis on each may vary.

Another area of conditioning and motor skill development is agility development. Specificity research tells us that agility development is highly specific to the sport or specific position within the sport. The authors recommend that coaches or athletes develop their own specific agility drills which are highly related to the sports skill to be practiced.

Aerobic Power
Anaerobic Power
Flexibility
Strength

FIGURE 1.3 *Sports Conditioning*

SUMMARY

There are many factors involved in successful athletic performance. The authors of this book have focused entirely on the physical conditioning involved in preparing for a sport. Athletes and coaches can greatly increase such abilities as aerobic and anaerobic power, muscular strength and endurance, and athletic power-speed-flexibility. The techniques can be used by athletes of both sexes and by a wide range of age groups.

For a more detailed description of the concepts introduced in this chapter, the reader is referred to the annotated references. In Chapter 2 we will deal with the scientific bases of athletic conditioning.

REFERENCES

1. Clarke, H. Harrison, ed. "Strength Development and Motor-Sports Improvement." *Physical Fitness Research Digest* 4 (October 1974): 1–17.
2. Cratty, Bryant J. *Movement Behavior and Motor Learning.* 3d ed. Philadelphia: Lea & Febiger, 1973.
3. Burke, Edmund J., ed. *Toward an Understanding of Human Performance.* 2d ed. Ithaca, NY: Mouvement Publications, 1981.
4. *Exercise and Sports Science Reviews*, vol. 1. Jack H. Wilmore, ed. New York: Academic Press, 1973.
5. Fox, Edward L. *Sports Physiology.* 2d ed. Philadelphia: W. B. Saunders Co., 1984.
6. Jensen, Clayne R., and Fisher, Garth A. *Scientific Basis of Athletic Conditioning.* 2d ed. Philadelphia: Lea & Febiger, 1979.
7. Knuttgen, Howard G. "Physical Conditioning and Limits to Performance." In R. H. Strauss, ed., *Sports Medicine and Physiology.* Philadelphia: W. B. Saunders Co., 1979, pp. 94–110.
8. O'Shea, John P. *Scientific Principles of Strength Fitness.* 2d ed. Reading, MA: Addison-Wesley, 1976.
9. Morehouse, Lawrence E. "Athletic Physiology." *Proceedings of the 4th National Conference on Medical Aspects of Sports.* AMA, November 25, 1962.
10. Stone, William J. "A Pre-Conditioning Program for Team Sports." *Arizona Prep.* 4 (May 1974): 18–20.
11. Stone, William J. "Sports Conditioning." *Osteopathic Annals* 9 (October 1981): 12–15, 18.
12. Taylor, Albert W. *The Scientific Aspects of Sports Training.* Springfield, IL: Charles C Thomas, 1975.
13. Wilmore, Jack H. *Training for Sport and Activity: The Physiological Basis of the Conditioning Process.* 2d ed. Boston: Allyn and Bacon, 1982.

2

Physiology of Fitness and Strength for Sports

In order to understand better the scientific bases of training and conditioning, a brief review of some physiological aspects of athletic performance is presented here. Special focus is aimed at the muscular system because the muscles are ultimately responsible for the movement and performance of the athlete. The descriptions are succinct so that the reader can move rapidly to succeeding chapters that make application of this information to training and conditioning techniques. Readers who require more detailed information should consult the references.

SPORTS FITNESS: AEROBIC AND ANAEROBIC MECHANISMS

Each time that an athlete moves—whether to run, jump, throw, kick, or produce any sports movement—the immediate source of energy at the muscle level is the high-energy phosphate compound adenosine triphosphate (ATP). The two major metabolic systems responsible for supplying ATP to the muscles are the aerobic and anaerobic pathways. The aerobic system supplies energy through a complex series of steps involving the Krebs cycle, the electron transport system, and the utilization of oxygen at the mitochondrial level in the muscle cell (fiber). The major sources of energy for the aerobic system include free fatty acids and carbohydrates. The anaerobic system bypasses the Krebs cycle in the absence of sufficient oxygen and utilizes carbohydrates as an energy source. The anaerobic system has the additional flexibility of releasing ATP through two different substrate mechanisms. One of these mechanisms relies on stored creatine phosphate (CP), while the others involves the production of high levels of lactic acid (LA).

Stage I. ATP-CP

Exercise physiologists have identified three energy-yielding mechanisms that encompass all sports activities. The three mechanisms differ in the amount or limits of ATP energy they can supply. Those limits are converted from quantitative amounts to time limits at maximal utilization rates for ease in discussing sports activities. The anaerobic (AN) Stage I mechanism comes into play in brief bursts of activity extending from fractions of a second to 15 seconds (Figure 2.1). Most sports skills are performed within that time span: bursting out of the blocks in a dash, throwing a ball, jumping for a rebound, and making a block or tackle. The energy is supplied by the ATP–CP mechanism at a very high rate for a very brief period. The ATP for this activity is readily stored in the muscle and is rapidly resynthesized with the aid of CP after use—thus the ability to repeat the act quickly or to repeat it after a brief rest.

Energy Mechanism	Sports Activity	Time Limitation	ATP Yield
I. (AN)ATP–CP	Brief bursts—e.g., 50-m dash, jumping, throwing, tackling	Up to 15 seconds	High rate, very limited
II. AN–LA	"All-out"—e.g., 400-m run, 100-m swim, repeated fast breaks	30–60 seconds	High rate, limited
III. AER	Continuous endurance—e.g., 5,000-m run, marathon, sports and games	Over 2 minutes	Low rate, "theoretically unlimited"

FIGURE 2.1 *Energy Mechanisms for Muscular Contraction*

Stage II. AN-LA

There are times when the athlete must extend himself or herself at a high rate for more than just a few seconds. As the athlete races around the quarter-mile track or engages in a series of fast breaks in basketball, an additional source of ATP can be supplied for a longer but definitely limited period (30-60 seconds). By utilizing carbohydrates directly, the AN–lactic–acid (LA) mechanism can produce larger amounts of ATP at a relatively high rate. The Stage II mechanism can be used at critical times in sport, but it has an extremely high aftercost. The by-product of the AN–LA mechanism is lactic acid and it is accompanied by a high level of oxygen debt if carried to its limit. Indeed, the athlete who has "burned it" in wind sprints or other Stage II activities can be left exhausted and require considerable time to recover. While metabolic recovery from Stage I activities will be nearly complete in three minutes, recovery from an all-out, Stage II effort may require an hour or more. All sports activities involve some aspect of AN Stage I, and AN activity is certainly associated with the more exciting aspects of sport. AN activity cannot continue for long, however, without the involvement of the aerobic system (AER).

Stage III. AER

Most sports entail fairly continuous periods of action punctuated with AN bursts. When activity continues beyond two minutes up to two hours or more, the Stage III mechanism is employed. Although the AER mechanism produces ATP energy at a very low rate, it is "theoretically unlimited."[5] The AN mechanisms have finite limits (Stage I) or LA tolerance limits (Stage II). The AER mechanism is a continuous cycle of ATP production and resynthesis. It is capable of tapping copious supplies of stored muscle glycogen and triglycerides as well as free fatty acids. The endurance activities, such as distance running and swimming and cross-country skiing, are usually associated with Stage III. The "cruising," dribbling, and constant movement in sports often make them very AER in nature. Soccer and basketball are excellent examples of sports with a large AER ingredient and significant AN action. AER power has been designated as the foundation of athletic conditioning. The ability to continue practicing or playing without undue fatigue and the ability to recover from vigorous activity are determined by the AER system. The ability to delay fatigue is also a significant factor in injury prevention.

As long as there are sufficient fuel (glycogen and free fatty acids) and oxygen available, the athlete can perform in a steady state. Steady state exercise means that the oxygen uptake meets the oxygen demands of the activity and little or no lactic acid buildup occurs in the muscles.

In the preceding chapter the *aerobic* power system was described as the ability of the athlete to continue performance without becoming prematurely fatigued. The aerobic capacity is determined by the ability of the body to deliver and take up oxygen into the tissue. This means a step-by-step process of 1) getting oxygen into the lungs (ventilation); 2) having the oxygen pass the membrane between the lungs and the blood to combine with hemoglobin, an O_2 carrying agent; 3) having the oxygenated blood pumped out to the muscles by the heart (cardiac output); and 4) getting the oxygen into the muscle tissues where it is needed (oxygen uptake). The last step involves sufficient blood vessels (capillaries) to carry oxygenated blood to the muscle fiber and then to the energy powerhouses (mitochondria) within the muscle tissue where oxygen is absorbed. All of these processes are improved by aerobic training.

The foregoing discussion relates to the three

mechanisms for supplying energy for muscle contraction. The three mechanisms will supply ATP either aerobically or anaerobically. The mechanisms are described graphically in Figure 2.1.

HIGH	Running — Swimming — Basketball
MEDIUM	Hockey — Football — Tennis — Volleyball
LOW	Baseball — Archery — Golf

FIGURE 2.2   *Aerobic Demands of Sports*

AER-AN TRAINING EFFECTS

Aerobic Training Effects

Repeated overload of the aerobic system results in numerous training effects within the various physiological systems. *Overload* simply means subjecting the systems or muscles to activity loads greater than those to which they are normally accustomed. Training effects are usually increases in the functional capacity or magnitude of the various systems that contribute to physical output. In the circulatory system the heart and blood vessels are much affected by training. The heart muscle becomes stronger and capable of greater output per minute (cardiac output). More blood vessels (capillaries) become available within the muscle, making easier the delivery of oxygen to the tissues. The blood volume and oxygen-carrying capacity (hemoglobin) increases, thus adding to the effect of more capillaries. The number and density of mitochondria increase in the cell, also increasing the oxygen uptake.

The respiratory system is also influenced by training and greater amounts of oxygenated air can be brought into the lungs (ventilation). The exchange of oxygen from the lungs to the blood and from the blood to the tissues is enhanced. The oxygen uptake increases, forestalling oxygen debt in the athlete. At less than maximum effort the athlete is capable of faster recovery when better trained. The combined result of increasing the capacity of the various systems operating in aerobic work is rather dramatic, resulting in the athlete's ability to perform at higher levels.

The aerobic demands of various sports are listed in Figure 2.2.

Anaerobic Training Effects

The anaerobic mechanisms are also affected by training but the exact scientific explanation of this phenomenon is not clear and may, in part, be due to psychological factors. ATP concentration, anaerobic enzymes, and myofibril density within the muscle are increased by anaerobic training. Athletes who undergo severe training programs have considerably greater tolerance for pain and discomfort than nonathletes. This indeed may be the hallmark of many champion athletes, i.e., their willingness to persevere at intense training levels and to give maximal effort in the latter stages of the game.

MUSCLE STRUCTURE AND CONTRACTION

The internal structure of the muscle can best be described by likening it to a huge telephone cable with thousands of wires packed tightly together but individually insulated and combined in clusters. In viewing the cross section of a muscle, it is apparent that there are thousands of fibers bound together by connective tissue, each with its individual insulation and nerve innervation. As few as ten and as many as several hundred fibers can contract together to form a *motor unit*. The motor unit is the smallest functioning unit of contraction within the muscle; i.e., the muscle tends to contract in units, a few or many, depending upon the demands on the muscle. The motor unit is composed of the motor nerve fiber, its branches, and all the muscle fibers they innervate. All of the fibers in a motor unit respond when the threshold is reached. Some motor units contract readily (low threshold), while others will contract only under vigorous stimulation from the nervous system (high threshold). Stimulation is carried from the brain to the muscle by the nervous system.

The method the nervous system uses to increase or decrease the strength of the contraction involves changes in the frequency of stimulation messages to the muscle. This results in the contraction of few or many motor units as the case may demand. Thus the athlete can produce maximum effort or fine movements with the same muscle or muscle groups.

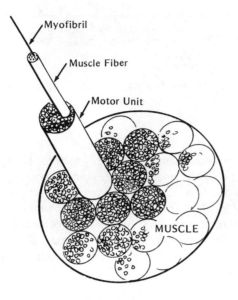

FIGURE 2.3 *Muscle Cross Section*

Muscle Fiber and Fiber Type

The basic element or cell of the muscle is called a *muscle fiber*. To gain some perspective of internal structure, it should be noted that the largest muscle fibers are about the size of a human hair. The fiber may run the entire length of the muscle but it is more likely to be linked in series within the belly of the muscle. (See Figure 2.4.)

One of the most fascinating discoveries relating to muscle physiology in athletes involves fiber typing work from muscle biopsies. Sections of muscle tissue are removed to determine the percentage of fast (white) or slow (red) twitch fibers within the muscle. Fast twitch fibers (FT) are high in glycogen (sugar), ATP supply, and predominate in high-speed and power activities. The FT fibers contract with great force, rapidly, but also fatigue quickly. The slow twitch fibers (ST) have a much greater blood vessel supply, oxidative capacity, and predominate in aerobic or endurance activities. ST fibers do not contract with great force but can sustain contractions for long periods. The type of fiber is apparently determined by the nervous system innervation, and some athletes will have a greater abundance of one type of fiber than of the other. (See Figure 2.5.)

A major concern for coaches and athletes is that aerobic training *does not* significantly train the fast twitch fibers and anaerobic training *does not* significantly train the slow twitch fibers. There is a tendency for some FT fibers to become more

oxidative with endurance training. Concentration on only one type of training may be sufficient if the sport requires only aerobic or anaerobic output but most team sports do not fall into only one category. Most team sports will require training of *both aerobic and anaerobic mechanisms* but in proportions that specifically match the demands.

Muscle Contraction

To understand how the muscle contracts, it is necessary to focus on the minute structures within the muscle fiber responsible for shortening the fiber. The myofibril is composed of alternating strips of myosin, a heavy protein filament, and actin, a thin, segmented protein filament. Columns of myofibrils pack the muscle fiber, running parallel with it. When the muscle is stimulated to contract, tiny hooks or "fingers" located on the myosin element reach across, link up with, and pull the actin strips past the myosin strips. This causes the fiber, and thus the muscle, to shorten. These "cross-bridges" are known as *micellae*, and their action produces a sliding effect as the actin filaments are drawn past the myosin filaments.

ATP has previously been described as the energy source for muscle contraction. Briefly, the muscle contracts after a message has come down from the brain via the nervous system and triggers ATP within the myofibril by a complex biochemical process. This ATP triggering results in myosin and actin coming together (muscle contraction).

Strength Training Effects

A number of physiological changes take place in the muscle when it is repeatedly subjected to an overload such as occurs with strength training. These changes involve the nervous pathways from the brain to the muscle, the tendonous attachments of the muscle, and the muscle itself. The combination of these changes can produce dramatic increases in strength and muscular endurance over a period of time.

Perhaps the earliest and yet most lasting effect of overloading the muscle involves the nervous system. The motor nerve pathways carrying messages from the brain to the muscle during specific strength-building exercises become so frequently and vigorously bombarded that there is an increase in the efficiency of travel along those routes. In

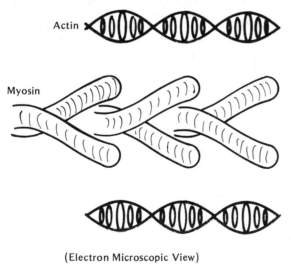

FIGURE 2.4 *Muscle Fiber*

Predominant Fiber Type	Sport Demands	Athletes
Fast Twitch (White)	Speed and power	Sprinters, weight lifters
Slow Twitch (Red)	Endurance activities	Distance runners, swimmers

FIGURE 2.5 *Fiber Type and Sports*

FIGURE 2.6 *Myofibril Structure*

motor skill development this change is associated with learning, and strength-building exercises are subject to the same changes. The strength builder "learns" the skill and mechanics of the strength-building exercise and the increased efficiency results in a more effective use of force. Perhaps a large portion of early strength gains represent greater efficiency in the application of force and nervous stimulations of high-threshold motor units not generally called upon to work.

Hypertrophy, or increase in size, occurs as the muscle is trained. The covering of the individual muscle fiber thickens and toughens as do the tendons supporting the muscle. This yields greater protection for the muscle and makes it less susceptible to injury. The increase in size is in no way proportional to increases in strength and muscular endurance. Barely measurable increases in size may accompany very great increases in strength and endurance. This effect needs to be emphasized because many athletes, both men and women, do not desire noticeable increases in muscle size.

As the muscle hypertrophies, the fibers grow larger rather than increasing in number. Much of the increase in size can be accounted for by increase in muscle sarcoplasm or fluid in the fiber. Increases in the total amount of stored glycogen and other chemicals involved in ATP production accompany the increase in fluid. The number and size of myofibrils (contractile protein) increase. Many small changes in the muscle and nervous systems add up to a dramatic increase in muscular strength.

SUMMARY

The physiology of fitness and strength is far more complex than is suggested in this brief chapter. Those who desire to gain more information regarding the physiology of exercise and sports are referred to the bibliography. A great deal is known about the physiology of exercise and especially training effects. In Chapter 3 we will describe some of the basic techniques used in conditioning for sports.

REFERENCES

1. Åstrand, Per-Olof, and Rodahl, Kaare. *Textbook of Work Physiology*. 2d ed. New York: McGraw-Hill, 1977.

2. Armstrong, Robert B. "Energy Release in the Extrafusal Muscle Fiber." *Neuromuscular Mechanisms for Therapeutic and Conditioning Exercises*, pp. 55–77. Baltimore: University Park Press, 1976.

3. Burke, Edmund J. "Work Physiology and the Components of Physical Fitness in the Analysis of Human Performance." *Toward An Understanding of Human Performance*. 2d ed. Ithaca, NY: Mouvement Publications, 1982.

4. deVries, Herbert. A *Physiology of Exercise for Physical Education and Athletics*. 3d ed. Dubuque, IA: William C. Brown Co., 1980.

5. Fox, Edward L. *Sports Physiology*. 2d ed. Philadelphia: W. B. Saunders Co., 1984.

6. Fox, Edward L., and Mathews, Donald K. *The Physiological Basis of Physical Education and Athletics*. Philadelphia: Saunders College Publishing, 1981.

7. Goldsmith, A. L., et al. "Mechanism of Work-Induced Hypertrophy in Skeletal Muscle." *Medicine and Science in Sports* 7 (1975): 185–198.

8. Gollnick, P. D., and Hermanson, L. "Biochemical Adaptations to Exercise: Anaerobic Metabolism." *Exercise and Sports Sciences Reviews*, vol. 1, pp. 1–43. New York: Academic Press, 1973.

9. Holloszy, John O. "Biochemical Adaptations to Exercise: Aerobic Metabolism." *Exercise and Sport Sciences Reviews*, vol. 1, pp. 45–71. New York: Academic Press, 1973.

10. Ianuzzo, C. David. "The Cellular Composition of Human Skeletal Muscle," *Neuromuscular Mechanisms for Therapeutic and Conditioning Exercises*, pp. 31–53. Baltimore: University Park Press, 1976.

11. Karlson, Jan. "Localized Muscular Fatigue: Role of Muscle Metabolism and Substrate Depletion." *Exercise and Sports Sciences Reviews*, vol. 7, pp. 1–42. Franklin Institute Press, 1979.

12. Krahenbuhl, Gary S. "Muscle Biopsy Research: Implications for Competitive Athletics." *Arizona Journal of Health, Physical Education, and Recreation* 20 (Fall 1976): 8–12.

13. MacDougall, J. D. et al. "Mitochondrial Volume Density in Human Skeletal Muscle Following Heavy Resistance Training." *Medicine and Science in Sports* 11 (1979): 164–166.

14. Taylor, A. W. "Endurance Training—Scientific Application." *The Scientific Aspects of Sports Training*, pp. 5–17. Springfield, IL: Charles C Thomas, 1975.

15. Thorstensson, Alf et al. "Muscle Strength and Fiber Composition in Athletes and Sedentary Men." *Medicine and Science in Sports* 9 (1977): 26–30.

16. Vrbová, Gerta. "Influence of Activity on Some Characteristic Properties of Slow and Fast Mammalian Muscles." *Exercise and Sport Sciences Reviews*, vol. 7, pp. 181–213. Franklin Institute Press, 1979.

17. Wenger, H. A. "The Physiology of Endurance Training." *The Scientific Aspects of Sports Training*, pp. 18–28. Springfield, IL: Charles C Thomas, 1975.

3

Aerobic and Anaerobic Conditioning

Training techniques for aerobic and anaerobic conditioning have reached a high level of sophistication. Some basic elements are essential for any training program if the program is to be effective. Those elements, along with the ones discussed in Chapter 4, form the basis for the programs offered in Part II for specific sports. There are several effective ways of training for aerobic and anaerobic conditioning. As long as the basic elements and the requirements of specificity are met, the training program will be effective.

A major contributor to the effectiveness of endurance and strength training is *overload*, which simply means continuously subjecting the athlete to work loads greater than those to which he or she is normally accustomed. In strength training, overload is accomplished primarily by increasing the resistance (weight). By progressively applying the basic elements of training, the aerobic and anaerobic systems are overloaded. The concepts of *progression* is discussed in more detail later in this chapter.

Chapters 3 (Aerobic and Anaerobic Conditioning), 4 (Strength Training for Sports), and 5 (Flexibility, Warm-Up, and Stretching) are intended to be used as detailed references for coaches and athletes using the programs enumerated in Part II. They describe the techniques involved in the programs designed by the authors for specific sports. Additional suggestions for implementing training programs are offered in Chapter 8 (The Conditioning Program: Putting It All Together). All aspects of sports conditioning could be included under the heading of either aerobic or anaerobic conditioning. Of the four target areas identified in Chapter 1 (anaerobic power, aerobic power, strength, and flexibility), both strength and flexibility training could be labeled anaerobic conditioning. Those two areas, however, have been treated in separate chapters and in some detail (Chapters 4 and 5).

BASIC ELEMENTS OF CONDITIONING

Three basic elements determine the effectiveness of sports fitness conditioning programs: 1) intensity, 2) duration, and 3) frequency. Regardless of the mode of training, these three elements will determine how well conditioned the athlete will become in a training program. This means that an athlete can produce good training effects by running, swimming, cycling, or any other whole body activity that can be done with some intensity for a selected period of time.

The whole body exercise most often used for training athletes in a wide variety of sports is running. There is good reason for this. Running does not require "learning," it can be done with a minimum expenditure of time, and it is more specific to most sports than other training modes. Most sports or games require the athlete to move around on the ground, so running is an easily adapted training technique. Naturally, swimmers, skaters, or cyclists would not train by running, since they can select the more specific training modes that suit their sports. Athletes occasionally resent the time spent in this type of conditioning, but running is really the most logical training mode for aerobic and anaerobic conditioning for a wide range of sports.

Intensity

In sports conditioning the degree to which the athlete works physically is a measure of the intensity of training. More intense training causes a more extreme response on the part of the body: the heart rate is higher, breathing is faster, oxygen debt is incurred earlier, and exhaustion occurs sooner. In running, swimming, or cycling, the *rate* at which one runs, swims, or cycles determines the intensity of training.

The two simplest means of gauging the intensity of sports conditioning are measuring the *time* it takes to run or swim a distance, and determining the athlete's HR (heart rate) at the conclusion of the activity. An example of two training bouts at different intensities for the same athlete would be:

Athlete	*Training* Mode	Distance	Time	HR	*Relative* Intensity
"A"	Running	¼ mi.	1:30	150	Lower
"A"	Running	¼ mi.	1:15	175	Higher

Similar examples could be given for many training modes: swimming, cycling, stair stepping, or other whole body activities. An important concept to note is that intensity will be *relative*. This means that for each athlete the work load imposed will lie on a continuum from low to high. It also means that another athlete, "B," might be better conditioned and respond with a *lower* HR for running the same distances at the same rate (time) as athlete "A." Although the two training bouts are less intense for athlete "B," one bout is still more intense than the other.

Athlete	*Training* Mode	Distance	Time	HR	*Relative* Intensity
"B"	Running	¼ mi.	1:30	125	Lower
"B"	Running	¼ mi.	1:15	150	Higher

The use of HR as a measure of intensity is based upon the concept that each athlete has a maximum heart rate (Max HR). To estimate Max HR, the following formula is used:

$$
\begin{array}{ll}
 & \textit{Example} \\
220 & 220 \\
\underline{-\text{ Age}} & \underline{-\ 20}\ (\text{Age}) \\
\text{Max HR} & 200\ (\text{Max HR estimated})
\end{array}
$$

Thus an eighteen-year-old athlete would have a *predicted* Max HR of 202. It should be noted that this is only an estimate and the true Max HR might vary by ± ten beats. To determine the HR necessary for training effect to take place, a percentage of the Max HR is used to determine the training heart rate (THR). Two techniques can be used and they are illustrated in Figure 3.1. For a training effect to take place the THR must reach 50–60 percent of Max HR. Athletes, who require intense training, will usually train at 80–95 percent of Max HR. The simplest technique would be to take an HR of 80–90 percent of the predicted Max HR, e.g., 90 percent of Max HR 200 = THR 180. An adjusted formula can also be used based upon the difference between the resting HR and the Max HR. The difference between these two is multiplied by 60–80 percent and *added* to the resting HR, e.g.,

$$
\begin{array}{lll}
\text{Step 1.} & \text{Max HR 200} & \\
 & \underline{-\ 60}\ \ (\text{Rest HR}) & \\
 & 140 & \\
 & \underline{\times\ 80\%} & \\
 & 112 & (80\%\ \text{of difference}) \\
 & & \\
\text{Step 2.} & 112 & \\
 & \underline{+\ 60}\ \ (\text{Rest HR}) & \\
 & 172 & \text{THR adjusted}
\end{array}
$$

This technique is more commonly used for determining THR for less fit adults. (See Figure 3.1.)

The intensity of an exercise can be quickly determined by palpating the carotid artery at the neck (just under the back corner of the jaw). The pulse will be very strong at that point after exercise and a *ten-second count immediately as exercise*

% Max	THR	Max HR (Min.)	Adjusted THR
95	190	200	174
90	180	200	168
80	160	200	156
60	120	200	132

FIGURE 3.1   *THR (Training Heart Rates)*
(Based upon Max HR 200 and Resting HR 60)

ends will closely estimate the exercise HR. The ten-second HR count is multiplied by six to convert to a one-minute count. (See Figure 3.2 for easy conversion.)

> *PRINCIPLE:* The more intense the training (whether aerobic or anaerobic) the greater the training effect. Duration can compensate for less intensity in aerobic conditioning.

Duration

Although intensity is a major element in training athletes, the duration of training will also influence the training effect. The *duration* of training refers to the length of time the athlete actually works during a training session. For example, an athlete may run for three minutes, rest for five minutes, and run again for three minutes. The duration of training is actually six minutes. In another session, an athlete may run continuously for six minutes duration but at a different intensity.

The objective of the training (aerobic or anaerobic) will determine the duration. Aerobic training is conducted at lower intensities but greater duration than anaerobic training. Since anaerobic training is of high intensity for brief periods, duration is accomplished by repeated bouts of activity in a training session.

> *PRINCIPLE:* The greater the duration of training (whether aerobic or anaerobic) the greater the training effect.

Frequency

The number of times per week that the athlete trains is the measure of frequency. Most school athletic teams practice five days per week. This is based on the five-day school week with weekends off. Some athletes may practice six, or possibly seven, days per week, while others may practice only three or four days per week. The practice referred to is primarily skills and strategy practice.

Physical conditioning also varies from team to team or athlete to athlete in terms of frequency. Conditioning frequency is greater in the early stages of training than in the later stages. For example, a team may be conditioned daily in the pre-season period but use only one to three days per week for maintaining condition during the season. Studies

10-sec. Count	HR (Min.)	10-sec. Count	HR (Min.)
35	210	25	150
34	204	24	144
33	198	23	138
32	192	22	132
31	186	21	126
30	180	20	120
29	174		
28	168		
27	162		
26	156		

FIGURE 3.2 *Heart Rate Counts*

on training effects indicate that significant levels of conditioning can be accomplished in the frequency range of two to four times per week. Less physically demanding sports may require only twice-a-week training sessions, while more physically demanding sports may require five or six training sessions per week.

A training program with a frequency of two to three times per week over a period of six to eight weeks is usually sufficient to produce significant training effects. Greater training effects require more frequency over a longer period of time. *Maintaining* sports fitness levels does not require as much frequency as it does to attain them. As few as one or two training sessions per week will maintain high percentages of sports fitness and strength over a sports season.

> *PRINCIPLE:* The frequency of physical training must fall in the two-to-four times per week range to produce training effects of value to the athlete.

Progression

Progression is also an important aspect of effective training. Progression is accomplished by gradually increasing the intensity and duration of training as the athlete becomes more physically fit. In strength training "progressive resistance" describes the overload on the muscles and there is a "progressive overload" for whole body conditioning. Over a period of time the athlete is able to tolerate higher work intensities for longer periods of time (duration). An example of a progressive increase for intensity could come from an earlier example:

Date	Athlete	Training Mode	Distance	Time
9/1	"A"	Running	¼ mi.	1:30
9/15	"A"	Running	¼ mi.	1:15

The example shows that athlete "A" was capable of running 1/4 mi. fifteen seconds faster on 9/15. The second bout of training was more intense, thus the example illustrates progression in training. A similar example could be given for progression in duration. The athlete may have run for a total of six minutes on 9/1 and ten minutes on 9/15.

In the early stages of training the athlete will not be able to tolerate the intensity and duration that can be handled later in the training season. The wise use of progression by the athlete or coach enables the athlete to reach an optimum level of condition for the sport in the most efficient way.

PRINCIPLE: The intensity and duration of physical training should be gradually and continually increased to reach optimum levels of sports fitness.

Interaction

There is an *interaction* between intensity, duration, and frequency, especially in aerobic training. This means that although intensity may be the primary overload factor, overload (and training effect) can also be achieved by increasing the duration and/or the frequency. The total amount of work done by the athlete may be the ultimate determinant of training. Greater amounts of work are accomplished by athletes in modern training programs. This is one of the most significant factors to account for better performance in track and swimming today when compared to past performances.

Athletes can compensate for training at lower intensity by working longer (duration) or more often (frequency). It should also be noted, however, that even endurance athletes, who focus on great duration and total work for a training effect, will also engage in high intensity training. The reason for this is to train also the high-threshold anaerobic fibers (FT) which can contribute to high-level aerobic performance.

CONTINUOUS TRAINING (AEROBIC)

The basic technique for developing aerobic fitness is low intensity *continuous* activity for periods of five minutes or longer. The duration of activity is progressively increased to ten to fifteen to twenty minutes or longer. The intensity is also progressively increased so that the athlete covers greater distances in the same time. Dr. Kenneth Cooper popularized aerobic training for adults by the publication of his best-selling book on aerobics. The beneficial effects of aerobic training are detailed in Chapter 2. As the capacities of circulatory, respiratory, and muscular systems increase, the ability to deliver oxygen to the muscle tissues increases. Anaerobic (lactic acid) energy use is delayed and fatigue is postponed as the athlete increases his or her aerobic power.

LSD

Continuous training has also been identified as long-slow-distance (LSD). This variation of continuous training involves greater *duration* and less intensity as a means of developing aerobic power. It is very effective in producing greater aerobic power. It is a classic example of the use of *duration* in training to compensate for lower intensity as discussed above.

An example of a continuous (aerobic) training regimen for one month might look like this:

July	Training Mode	Distance	Goal/Min.	Times/ Week
Week 1	Run	1.0 mi.	8:00	3
Week 2	Run	1.5 mi.	12:00	3
Week 3	Run	1.5 mi.	11:30	3
Week 4	Run	2.0 mi.	15:00	3

In the example the duration of training has increased from 1.0 mi. to 2.0 mi. and from 8:00 to 15:00 min. The *intensity* has also increased because the rate of running the first week was 8:00 min. for 1.0 mi., while in week 4 the rate has increased to 7:30 min. for 1.0 mi. The latter figure is based on running 2.0 mi. in 15:00 min.

Over a period of time endurance athletes will develop great duration in their training until they are running twice a day and covering more than 100 miles in training per week.[5] This means that they will run at least six miles in each session.

Marathon runners may run as much as 150 miles per week in preparation for an event which is estimated to be 99 percent aerobic.

Fartlek

Another variation of continuous training is called *Fartlek*. The athlete runs continuously to train aerobic capacity but varies the intensity during the training session. As the athlete feels the need to rest, the intensity is reduced, and when the athlete feels recovered the intensity is increased for a period of time.

There is relatively little technique to be learned when running for continuous training. Perhaps the major exception for most athletes is concentrating on running "flat-footed." This means that an athlete who is used to landing on the sole of the foot when running must remember to land on the heel, then sole.

Fartlek training points out the variation in intensity that can occur in aerobic training. Aerobic training can progress from very light activity to high-intensity aerobic training which also involves the anaerobic system, specifically Stage II or AN-LA. This implies that, at some point, the athlete has crossed over from aerobic work to anaerobic work.

THE ANAEROBIC THRESHOLD

In Chapter 2 the various energy systems are discussed and treated as independent entities. That concept implies that the athlete works either in aerobic metabolism or in anaerobic metabolism. Although most sports movements require energy predominately from Stage I (ATP-CP), or Stage II (AN-LA), or Stage III (AER), there can be some overlap. Aerobic and anaerobic metabolism can be going on at the same time. In running 400m all out, the athlete is working primarily in Stage II (AN-LA), but Stage III (AER) is also engaged. The athlete is taking in oxygen, although not enough, during the period of the race. Conversely, a middle distance runner, who is performing a predominately AER effort, can be producing some LA because the intensity of the work has crossed over the anaerobic threshold (AT).

The concept of AT suggests that at some point, LA (lactic acid) begins to accumulate in the muscle tissue and then in the blood. That point is generally identified as a certain percentage of the athlete's maximum oxygen uptake or maximal AER power. A considerable research effort has been made to determine the AT. Training appears to raise the AT for the athlete, and well-trained athletes have a higher AT. Skinner[14] has suggested that there may be three phases in the transition from AER to AN work. These phases would include: 1) a period from low level to moderate AER work which is truly AER, 2) a second phase (40-60 percent of maximum oxygen uptake) when a small amount of LA begins to appear and has been labeled AT by some, and 3) a third phase from 65-90 percent of maximal oxygen uptake when LA increases significantly but the athlete can continue to work for prolonged periods. Above this level the AN-LA system is fully engaged and the athlete will exhaust in a very short time, probably less than a minute.

It is important for coaches and athletes to know that many sports and many athletic efforts involve both the aerobic and the anaerobic systems. Often the athlete must work for prolonged periods in the third phase of the AT (65-90 percent maximum). When the athlete must train for such an energy expenditure, or for some mixture of aerobic and anaerobic effort, the training involves the use of the interval technique.

INTERVAL TRAINING

Over the past several decades interval training has had a major impact on sports training. *Interval training* is alternating work and rest periods during a training session. Continuous training involves continuous work, which concludes the training session when it comes to an end. In interval training a work bout is followed by a rest period, then another work bout, and so on. The technique is credited to Dr. Woldemer Gerschler of Germany.[1] He introduced the technique about 1930 and it began to appear in the United States in the 1950s. A Finnish athlete named Pihkala used interval training in the early 1900s but the great Czech, Emil Zatopek, was the first to employ interval training seriously.[1]

Interval training rests on the very sound physiological fact that the athlete can produce a much greater total work load in a training session if the bouts of exercise are spaced. Astrand[2] found that a pace (intensity) that caused exhaustion in nine minutes could be continued for an hour. and much more work could be done if rest intervals were included:

Continuous	Interval
9 min. = 1,940 kg (work done)	1 hour = 64,800 kg
Max. HR = 204	Max. HR = 150
LA = 150 mg	LA = 20 mg

In this example the total work done in over an hour (on a bicycle) was *thirty-three times greater* than the continuous activity that caused exhaustion in nine minutes, yet the rate of work was the same. The Max. HR reached in nine minutes of continuous activity was 204 and the lactic acid level (LA) was 150 mg. Both of these figures signal the approach of exhaustion for persons exercising. The heart rate (150) and LA level (20 mg) for the interval technique are in the training zone but not close to the exhaustion level. An indication of how the HR responds during continuous and interval training is described in Figure 3.3.

It is possible to manipulate several factors in an interval training program to produce an overload. A basic interval training program might be designed as follows:

Distance	Rate	Rest	No. of Reps	Frequency
440 yds.	75 sec.	90 sec.	10	4 days

In this example the athlete runs 440 yards in 75 seconds, then rests for 90 seconds. At each training session this work-rest ratio is repeated ten times (ten reps), and there are four training sessions per week. An overload could be applied to the athlete by increasing the rate (from 75 to 70 sec.), by decreasing the rest (from 90 to 80 sec.), or by increasing the number of repeat intervals (ten to twelve reps). Thus, a later version of the interval program would be as follows:

Distance	Rate	Rest	No. of Reps	Frequency
440 yds.	70 sec.	80 sec.	12	4 days

Another interval training technique used by some coaches and athletes involves HR as a measure of intensity. A training HR (THR) is set at 160–180. (See Figure 3.1.) When this rate is reached, the athlete maintains the THR for a set period, then begins a rest interval until the HR recovers to 120–140. Recovery is not "complete" but the athlete is sufficiently recovered to work again soon at a high rate without reaching exhaustion such as occurs when training is carried on continuously to fatigue.

Another advantage of the interval training technique is that the athlete can work at very intense anaerobic rates (maximum) for brief periods of time. These repeated efforts produce an anaerobic training effect. Perhaps of even greater importance, these bouts of exercise exceed the intensity of play in most sports but prepare the athlete for those intense periods when they do occur in competition.

There are many ways of manipulating the

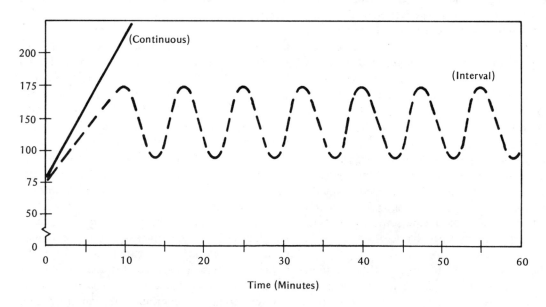

FIGURE 3.3 *Continuous vs. Interval Training*

work and rest intervals in interval training.[1] These variations of the internal technique have a variety of names aimed at developing quantity (many intervals at submaximal effort) or quality (maximal effort intervals). There can be an interaction among work, rest, and repetitions in the interval technique just as was observed with intensity, duration, and frequency in continuous training.

Although the interval between work bouts is identified as REST, the athlete is actually active at a reduced rate. At a minimum output, athletes should continue walking between work bouts and most athletes can jog easily. The cardiovascular system is still under stress during the rest period. Recovery, especially from lactic acid accumulation, is hastened by mild activity. Coaches and athletes have known this fact instinctively by the use of walking or jogging after wind sprints or other vigorous activity.

Aerobic and Anaerobic Intervals

Some general guidelines should be kept in mind when training for aerobic or anaerobic intervals. If the reader will recall the three mechanisms for supplying energy (see Figure 2.2), the kind of training interval should match as closely as possible the demands of the sport. Astrand[3] and others[4, 12] have recommended general training intervals for aerobic and anaerobic power. The basic intervals for conditioning the three energy mechanisms are summarized in Figure 3.4. Intervals below 20 seconds of work result in little LA accumulation, quick recovery, and can be repeated many times. The ATP-CP system has very rapid recovery, approaching full recovery in three minutes. Intervals at 30 seconds will result in significant increases in LA, and as the interval reaches 60 seconds, LA accumulation will maximize and recovery is greatly prolonged. A rest interval of four to five minutes

is necessary to yield sufficient recovery to sustain repeated AN-LA intervals. AN-LA training is very exhausting, both physically and mentally. The coach or athlete must "flirt" with the tolerance levels of this system or the training session can come to an abrupt halt at maximum oxygen debt. This means that the upper limits of LA tolerance have been achieved, and the athlete is exhausted. A small reduction (3.3 percent) in running speed has been found to drop the percentage of effort in terms of maximal oxygen uptake from 100 percent to 90 percent.[12]

The reader should be aware that these intervals are guidelines and are not intended to apply to each specific sports training program. They are, however, effective in guiding the coach or athlete to select aerobic or anaerobic intervals that match the energy output demands of the sport.

It should also be noted that there are some "gaps" in the intervals suggested in Figure 3.4. Those areas represent transition areas between the various Stages. For specific events or sports some intervals may need to be used within those transition areas.

The concept of AER intervals may appear at first to be a misnomer. Typically we consider continuous work to be the major technique for developing AER power, and intervals to be restricted to anaerobic training. The concept of AT (anaerobic threshold), however, suggests that some AER effort must be done at high work loads, which may also engage the AN system. Continuous AER training is usually carried on at 60–80 percent of maximum capacity. AER intervals, however, can train the athlete at 80 percent or above, which aids the athlete in peaking for AER power. AER intervals also fit more readily into the regular practice session than, for example, a 60-minute run. The highly conditioned endurance athlete will be capable of maintaining high intensity (80–90 percent) activity for prolonged periods (30–60 minutes). Such work is really continuous, but at an intensity

	Work	% Max	Rest	Reps
		ANAEROBIC		
ATP-CP	5–15 secs.	100	15 secs.–2 mins.	5–20
AN-LA	30–60 secs.	90	4–5 mins.	5–10
		AEROBIC		
Continuous	10–60 mins.	60–80	NA	1
AER Interval	3–5 mins.	80	3–5 mins.	3–10

FIGURE 3.4 *AN–AER Training Intervals*

that most athletes could tolerate only in shorter intervals.

Interval training techniques can be used to train all three energy supply systems: 1) ATP (Anaerobic), 2) Aerobic, and 3) Anaerobic (lactic acid). By using interval training, athletes in running and swimming events pile up staggering amounts of work in each practice session. Athletes in many sports can also gain the benefits of systematic training specifically geared to the demands of their sport. Training programs for specific sports are described in detail in Part II.

CIRCUIT TRAINING

Circuit training is a simple, efficient method of training that has been adopted by many coaches. It is a series of exercises that can be easily designed for a specific sport. Perhaps the greatest advantage of circuit training for sports is that *all aspects of physical conditioning* can be built into the circuit. The circuit can be designed to condition for *muscular strength* and *endurance, aerobic power, anaerobic capacity* or *speed,* and *flexibility.*

A circuit can be set up indoors or outdoors with a series of exercises to be completed in as short a period of time as possible. An athlete could do a number of push-ups, then move on to the next station and do several sit-ups, continuing through the entire series of exercises. A circuit might contain from six to twelve stations according to the need of the coach or athlete. (See Figure

3.5 for an example of a general conditioning circuit.)

Normally, a circuit is completed three times in a conditioning session but it could be run only once or twice if time must be saved. An overload is applied by increasing the number of times each exercise is done or by adding weight for weight training exercises. The time allowed to complete the circuit can also be reduced to increase the intensity of the training.

It is evident from Figure 3.5 that the coach or athlete can design circuits for a specific sport using as many exercises as time permits. The coach or athlete can concentrate the exercises on the specific needs of the sport, e.g., flexibility, arm strength, or leg power. Examples of specific circuits for various sports are listed in Part II.

SUMMARY

The three basic elements of conditioning programs are intensity, duration, and frequency. A progressive overload is applied to training by the use of the basic elements. Training goals can be accomplished through a variety of modes, such as running, swimming, cycling, or other whole body activities.

Continuous training is used primarily for aerobic conditioning, while interval training can be used to train both the aerobic and anaerobic systems. Circuit training is an efficient and effective

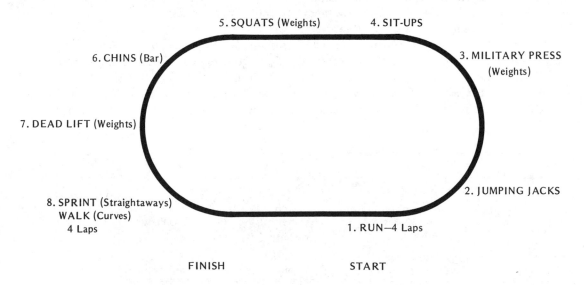

FIGURE 3.5 *Circuit Training: Set Up on a ¼-Mile Track*

technique for combining aerobic and anaerobic training, muscular strength and endurance, and flexibility.

REFERENCES

1. "A Positive Interval Addition to Speed." *Runners World*, June 1978, pp. 70–79.
2. Astrand, I. et al. "Intermittent Muscular Work." *Acta Physiol. Scand.* 48 (1960): 448.
3. Åstrand, Per-Olof, and Rodahl, Kaare. *Textbook of Work Physiology.* 2d ed. New York: McGraw-Hill, 1977.
4. Cooper, Kenneth H. *The Aerobics Way.* New York: M. Evans, 1977.
5. Costill, David L. *A Scientific Approach to Distance Running.* Track and Field News, 1979.
6. Daniels, Jack et al. *Conditioning for Distance Running.* New York: John Wiley & Sons, 1978.
7. Fox, Edward L., and Matthews, Donald K. *Interval Training: Conditioning for Sports and General Fitness.* Philadelphia: W. B. Saunders Co., 1974.
8. Fox, Edward L. *Sports Physiology.* 2d ed. Philadelphia: W. B. Saunders Co., 1984.
9. Karlsson, J. et al. "Training the Oxygen Transport System in Man." *J. Appl. Physiol.* 22 (1967): 1061.
10. Londeree, Ben R. "Anaerobic Threshold Training." *Toward An Understanding of Human Performance,* pp. 15–16. Ithaca, NY: Mouvement Publications, 1977.
11. Morgan, R. E., and Adamson, G. T. *Circuit Training.* London: Bell & Sons, 1961.
12. Peronnet, François, and Ferguson, Ronald J. "Interval Training." *The Scientific Aspects of Sports Training,* pp. 31–41. Springfield, IL: Charles C Thomas, 1975.
13. Pollack, Michael L. "The Quantification of Endurance Training Programs." *Exercise and Sport Sciences Review* 1, 73–102. New York: Academic Press, 1973.
14. Skinner, James S., and McClellan, Thomas H. "The Transition from Aerobic to Anaerobic Metabolism." *Research Quarterly* 51 (March 1980): 234–248.
15. Stone, William J. "Sports Conditioning." *Osteopathic Annals* 9 (October 1981): 12–15, 18.

4

Strength Training for Sports

This chapter provides the fundamental concepts and the specific information necessary to carry out a successful year-round strength training program for athletes. In order to do this, the reader must have a clear understanding of: the difference between strength training for athletes and other types of weight training; some terminology used in strength training; the essentials of strength training for athletes; the practical methods of varying the elements of intensity, duration, and frequency in the strength program; and the techniques of performing each pertinent strength exercise.

To be successful the strength training program should achieve two main objectives: 1) it must be effective in reducing the number of athletic injuries which could otherwise occur, and 2) it must be effective in improving athletic performance. The strength programs offered in Part II are based on the information developed in this chapter, and are directed toward achieving these two objectives.

TYPES OF WEIGHT TRAINING

The general subject of weight training has, in the past, been surrounded by misconceptions, inaccuracies, and misunderstanding. The reason for this is a general lack of knowledge about the use of weights in the specialized area of strength training for athletes. An understanding of the differences between strength training for athletes and the other types of weight training can help clarify the areas of misconception. Therefore,

each of the various types of weight training will be defined.

Rehabilitation

Resistance training is used widely as a clinical means of rehabilitating people with injuries. Chapter 6 will discuss injury prevention and rehabilitation in detail.

Bodybuilding

This type of training is generally associated with the physique (as with Mr. America or Mr. Universe competitions). The goals of the bodybuilder are a massive musculature, with beautiful, well-proportioned, and well-defined muscles. There are many professional and amateur bodybuilding competitions. Strength, power, muscular endurance, cardiovascular endurance, flexibility, agility, speed, or other athletic qualities are not essential for these competitions.

The bodybuilder usually works many repetitions on one isolated body part in order to enlarge the muscle by pumping the blood into it continuously. In some bodybuilding systems (blitz systems) circuits of several exercises on a single body part are performed over long periods of time. The result of this type of training is large but not necessarily strong muscles. With most bodybuilders, flexibility and agility are not included in the goals of their weight training; therefore they are susceptible to reduced flexibility and athletic ability.

Weight Lifting

There are two types of competitive weight lifting: Olympic Lifting and Power Lifting, and international and world competitions in both sports. The Olympic Lifts are included in the Olympic Games. In both Olympic Lifting and Power Lifting competition is conducted in the same manner. There are three judges for each event or "lift." Three attempts are allowed in each lift. One successful attempt in each lift is necessary to stay in the competition. The weight on the bar is increased in a manner similar to raising the high jump or pole vault bar. It is increased only once for each lift, until all lifters have made three attempts. If a lift is missed on the first or second attempt, the lifter may use the same weight for the next attempt. This attempt must be done within three minutes if no other lifters are going to attempt the same weight. The alternative is to attempt a heavier weight successfully in order to stay in the competition. The rules in both sports stipulate the strictest of form, and any variation is call for disqualifying the attempt. The winner is determined by the highest total poundage of the best attempt in each lift.

The *Olympic Lifts* are the "snatch" and the "clean and jerk." When done properly, they are extremely quick, athletic movements, unlike the Power Lifts. In the "snatch" the bar is lifted from the floor overhead in one movement. The "squat style" or "split style" may be used. The "clean and jerk" entails two movements: taking the bar from the floor to the shoulders (the clean), and thrusting it overhead, extending the arms (the jerk). The Military Press was one of the Olympic Lifts until the early 1970s.

Power Lifting consists of the Squat, the Bench Press, and the Dead Lift. More weight can be used in the Power Lifts, consequently they are done at slower speed than the very quick Olympic Lifts.

In the starting position for the *Squat*, the lifter has the barbell on his back and is standing erect. The line or midpoint of the thighs must drop until it breaks the imaginary plane parallel to the floor. The lifter then rises from this position again to the starting position. During the *Bench Press*, the bar is lowered to the chest, paused for one second, and raised again. The *Dead Lift* is performed by lifting the barbell from the floor until the body is standing completely erect, the weight held with the arms extended downward. The training for both Olympic and Power Lifting is extremely specialized and specific to the movements involved, and obviously concentrates mainly on developing maximum strength.

General Conditioning

Many persons use weight training as a means of keeping physically trim at every age. There are probably as many systems of training for this purpose as there are individuals participating in weight training to keep in shape. The public in the United States spends millions of dollars each year for spas, health clubs, YMCAs, and individually owned weights. With the acceptance of supplemental weight training programs for nearly every sport, many former athletes who used weight training for strength development continue to use it as a method of keeping physically trim. This is one of the side benefits offered the athlete by the inclusion of weight training in the athletic program. Weight training for such purposes does not replace aerobic training for cardiovascular conditioning.

Strength Training for Athletes

The term *strength* training rather than *weight* training for athletes is used since the goal is to develop strength by many different methods, and in many cases various machines, pulleys, and devices are used that employ no weights. In recent years active scientific study and widespread practical application of strength training by athletes and coaches throughout the world have shown conclusively that strength training can be extremely effective in improving athletic performance and preventing athletic injuries, if the proper type of strength program is employed.

The correct strength training program can offer the athlete increased speed, quickness, muscular endurance, coordination, explosive power, and flexibility, as well as pure strength. The most important concept to remember is that the correct type of strength program must be used in order to receive the specific results desired.

One of the old misconceptions concerning weight training was that it caused "muscle boundness" or loss of flexibility. Many scientific studies over a long period of time have shown that weight training does not impair flexibility and that it may, in fact, actually increase flexibility.[34, 13, 14] The proper training techniques, which nearly always include a full *"range of motion,"* are necessary to ensure that flexibility is maintained as a result of a weight training program.

Another misconception is that weight training causes slowed movement in the trained muscles. Studies conducted decades ago by Chui[6] and Karpovich and Zorbas[36] discounted this idea, and later research efforts have supported those results.[7] There is also evidence that an increase in muscular speed may accompany an increase in muscular strength.[7] The essential components and concepts of weight training for athletics are included in the following sections.

STRENGTH TRAINING TERMINOLOGY

Isometric Contraction

This type of muscle contraction involves no joint movement. Isometrics are usually done by applying pressure to an immovable object, but may be done by simply contracting the muscles while holding the limbs still. Isometric training was a popular form of strength building for sports during the early 1960s. The greatest amount of force can be achieved in an isometric contraction. The value of the strength developed is only effective in a narrow range close to the point at which it was developed. This major disadvantage has led to a limited use of isometrics for sports.

Isotonic Contraction

This type of muscle contraction involves limb or body movement. Although isotonic contraction for training is done against resistance, all movements of the body are technically isotonic movements, although some are not done against resistance. There are several types of isotonic contractions:

Concentric contraction involves shortening of the contracting muscle, which moves the resistance. The muscle overcomes the resistance, moving the limb through the motion by shortening itself.

Eccentric contraction entails lengthening of the muscle. This is done when a weight is lowered through the range of motion. The muscle slowly yields to the resistance, allowing itself to be stretched.

Isokinetic contraction is a special type of isotonic contraction. It is created by controlling the speed of the contraction mechanically. The purpose is to allow a maximal contraction to be achieved throughout the entire movement (range of motion). The maximal force that can be achieved at any one point in the movement varies. The speed of movement also influences force. The slower the isokinetic movement, the greater the amount of force that can be applied through the movement. It should be noted that during isokinetic movement the isokinetic device is set at a given speed. No matter how hard the individual attempts to force the device through the movement, the speed remains constant. The device includes a gauge that records the amount of force produced. With conventional isokinetic devices this includes a "needle type" indicator showing the amount of force currently being produced. The final reading shows the maximum amount of force produced at the peak of the contraction.

The majority of muscular contractions used in athletics are "explosive" in nature. As discussed in Chapter 1, power is developed when acceleration of an object is occurring in a brief time span. The amount of force behind this acceleration also determines the amount of power generated. Some athletic movements are composed of a coordinated chain of muscular contractions. These movements can use the summation of the forces developed by each succeeding contraction to create a greater amount of power and/or velocity. To improve performance of such movements it is advantageous to be able to imitate natural athletic movements at slightly slower speed against resistance. This is often done with pulleys, isokinetic equipment, weights, or other specially designed devices.

Variable resistance refers to a type of isotonic strength training equipment that changes the amount of resistance offered throughout the range of motion. The equipment is normally designed to offer resistance that closely matches the strength available throughout the movement.

Repetition is the completion of one entire cycle of an exercise. If an athlete does ten push-ups, he or she has done ten repetitions. (Repetitions is many times abbreviated "reps.") One repetition of the maximum weight that can be lifted is abbreviated 1RM (or 1 repetition maximum). It follows that "3RM" means "the highest weight with which three repetitions can be performed." The same is true for abbreviating any other repetition maximum. After the point where no more repetitions can be completed, momentary failure, or acute muscle fatigue (AMF) is experienced.[33]

Set is the completion of one "turn" or "bout." It can also be defined as a consecutive series of reps. If an athlete does ten push-ups and then rests, and then does ten again, he or she has done two sets of ten repetitions.

FACTORS INFLUENCING STRENGTH TRAINING

The basic factors and fundamental concepts of physical training which apply to all of the types of weight training include: the use of proper technique, the equipment available, which exercises are performed, diet, amount of sleep, rate of metabolism, body type, muscular makeup, injury history, psychological profile, environment, motivational factors, the variation of intensity, duration and frequency, and others.

In some instances these factors can be easily controlled and in other cases they cannot be controlled at all. The fact that so many variables exist is one reason for much of the confusion about weight training in general. The authors recognize the limitations inherent in individual situations on available workout time, space, equipment, transportation, participation in other sports, and other financial and physical considerations. The information that follows provides the reader with an organized approach to controlling as many of these factors as the situation permits.

ESSENTIALS OF STRENGTH TRAINING FOR ATHLETES

An understanding of the essentials of strength training for athletes represents the *first step* toward unraveling the misconceptions and confusion mentioned earlier. Each of the other four types of weight training is a separate "area of concentration." Each has its own goals, programs, exercises, training techniques, and methods. Ideas from each area have been successfully applied in athletes' strength programs but, despite this, some of the procedures and techniques used in each of these areas do not apply and should not be used in training athletes. It is necessary to be able to determine which ideas can be applied successfully to this type of training. The scientific research literature

in physical education indicates at least *six* essentials that should be present in an athlete's strength program. Each of the six has a substantial amount of documentation supporting it. The existence of these essentials therefore forms a scientific basis upholding and giving validity to the field of strength training for athletics.

By ascertaining whether or not these essentials are present one can determine if the strength program is fundamentally sound. In this way they can serve as a guideline to the athlete and the coach in creating, adjusting, and administering strength programs for athletes. Most important, a working knowledge of the essentials can ensure (by scientific support) that the strength program will produce positive results in achieving the athletes' two major objectives: preventing injuries and improving athletic performance.

The following are considered "The Essentials of Strength Training for Athletes":

1. Total Body

Each major body part needs to be included in all strength programs for athletes. This is necessary in order to improve athletic performance and to help prevent injuries. The proportional development of the muscle groups throughout the body ensures that the newly acquired muscular strength can become "functional strength." This is mainly true of athletic movements that require the transfer of force from one body part to another (i.e., the application of the principle of the summation of forces or the conservation of angular momentum). Overall development gives the athlete the capability of learning new skills more easily. The strengthening of the total body also helps to prevent athletic injuries. This occurs in two ways, the first being that stronger body parts are less likely to be injured. Strengthening all of the body parts eliminates weak areas especially vulnerable in heavy contact sports like football. Second, strengthening the total body in the proper way helps to eliminate injuries caused by muscular imbalance.

2. Progressively Increasing Overload

In order to develop maximum strength the athlete must use progressively increasing resistance. Strength training is perhaps the best example of the application of the "Overload Principle." To develop maximum strength, this principle is applied in the following way:

a) There must be an organized method of gradually increasing the resistance used in the strength exercises.
b) The completion of the sets and repetitions in the strength program must require maximum efforts.
c) Maximum strength is best developed by training heavy repetitions of 1–8 RM.

3. Stretching

Stretching is an extremely important essential in strength training for athletes, if only for the purpose of developing and maintaining the flexibility necessary in athletics. This means that athletes who are involved in a strength training program need to be involved in stretching exercises for the whole body on a daily basis. Besides flexibility, stretching has many other benefits. (See Chapter 5.) In fact, stretching *is* strength training. Consider the following:

a) When a muscle is placed on stretch, it is at its strongest position. The farther it can be stretched, the stronger it is.
b) The strongest muscular contraction comes following a pre-stretch. Some strength training systems such as "The Jones System" make active use of this principle.
c) Since stretching increases flexibility, the range of motion through which the body part can be moved is lengthened. It is therefore capable of increasing velocity over a greater distance, thereby creating greater force.

Considerable research confirms that stretching exercises increase flexibility. Research continues to present conflicting evidence as to whether or not weight training reduces or increases flexibility.[34] Some research studies indicate that, after 12 years of age, a person tends to become less flexible in some ways, unless he or she performs stretching exercises. There has never been a research study indicating that weight training, when combined with stretching exercises, reduces flexibility. In fact, studies have shown that strength training and stretching significantly increase sprint speed as well as flexibility.[13, 14]

4. Practicing the Sports Skills

Athletes need to perform the skills in their particular sport on a year-round basis. This practice is particularly essential when the off-season strength program is being performed. The reason for this was expressed by Sparrow,[21] a specialist in motor learning at the University of Illinois:

> It is often observed that following off-season weight training an athlete shows a fall-off in sport skill performance. This may be due to interference [3] from weight training during the non-competition period. To help reduce this performance decrement many athletes combine off-season conditioning with skill practice. Traditionally, due to the nature of the activity, team-sport athletes are unable to practice many of their particular skills during the off-season. Unfortunately, there is little experimental evidence that weight training itself produces physiological or psychological changes which actively inhibit skill performance. Typically, however, an athlete who does not follow a weight training or skill practice program during the off-season shows less reduction in performance than the regular weight trainer. Therefore, it seems likely that weight training is responsible for poor early season performance if not combined with skill practice. On the basis of these findings it is strongly recommended that off-season weight training be combined with a program of specific sport skill practice whenever possible. (For other sources supporting this statement, see [12, 18] and [24] in the bibliography.)

The skills should be performed in the normal way, that is, without any extra resistance. During the off-season strength program this should be done three or four days a week. A short five- to ten-minute period is all that is necessary to keep the skill pattern grooved.

Strength training for athletes utilizes the "Principle of Specificity" in terms of the application of two other essentials. These are applied mainly during the pre-season and in-season strength programs.

5. Specificity in Terms of Muscular Endurance

Strength training should be specific to the muscular endurance requirement of the sport. For example, a basketball player should generally do more repetitions in strength training than a shot-putter or even a football player because the amount of muscular endurance required in basketball is greater. Most sports require repeated bursts of activity, which challenge muscular endurance. The lower repetitions (1–8) used to develop maximum strength [4] in the off-season do not develop strength with the component of high endurance. The strength developed at low endurance can help the athlete perform with increased strength at high endurance. To accomplish this, the athlete must undergo a two- to three-week "adjustment phase" where lighter resistance is used at the desired endurance. This is usually done during the pre-season period.

6. Specificity in Terms of Range of Motion

The athlete's strength program during the pre-season and in-season periods should utilize, to a great extent, exercises that imitate the exact range of motion required in the sport. Exercises used to maintain strength in the large "power muscles" and exercises used to prevent injuries in key areas should also be utilized. However, all other strength exercises done at this time should be employed to improve performance through the specific range of motions that the activity requires. It has long been recognized in the area of motor learning that the specificity of a skill is distinct and peculiar to itself. Since the strength and power of athletic movements are developed specifically, having power in one movement does not guarantee having power in another.

In normal practice most coaches and athletes know that the exact range of motion must be used. Differences in ROM (range of motion) between training and actual performance in delicate, complex movements may result in no beneficial effects, and in fact may actually interfere with normal movement patterns. In strength training the greatest usable strength will be developed if the exact range of motion is followed. For example, if an athlete is training to strengthen the throwing motion, he needs to consider whether he is training to throw a football or to pitch a baseball. The movement in his strength program is then constructed to match the exact range of movement of the athletic skill as closely as possible. In the case of the throwing motion a wall pulley, Mini-Gym, or another similar device is often used.

7. Specificity in Terms of Speed of Movement

It is the opinion of the authors that specificity in terms of speed of movement should be employed in pre-season and in-season strength programs for athletes. We believe that the current scientific evidence supports this practice; however, there remains some controversy on this point within the field.

The major argument against strength training at fast speed involves the question of safety. Research on either side of the discussion remains scant. This is not to minimize the importance of safety—safety is definitely a factor that should be considered a major priority in the strength program and at all other times. (See Safety, p. 00.)

In most athletic activities high speed is a critical factor. The authors believe that the research surrounding "The Principle of Specificity," and in particular speed of movement, indicates that the strength training for athletics should be performed at high speed if the skill is performed at high speed. The slow speed strength developed by resistance training is primarily transferable to athletic movement only at the slower speed at which it was developed.[25] High speed resistance training should be done in the pre-season program as a means of transferring the slow speed strength developed in the off-season to the high speed requirement of the sport.

THE VARIABLE ELEMENTS (INTENSITY, FREQUENCY, DURATION)

When discussing strength training for athletes, it should be remembered that strength training is one of four types of conditioning for athletes. Therefore, the same elements that apply to aerobic and anaerobic conditioning also apply to strength training. These elements (intensity, duration, and frequency) are discussed in Chapter 3 in relation to aerobic and anaerobic training. As mentioned earlier in this chapter, strength training and stretching are actually special types of anaerobic conditioning. Circuit strength training is sometimes used for the development of aerobic conditioning. There is rarely a clear-cut distinction between aerobic and anaerobic exercise, since most activities are a blend of both systems.[34] For this reason, one cannot state that strength training is not sometimes aerobic; however, few if any research studies have shown circuit strength training to produce a significant cardiovascular training effect. In any case, the effects produced by strength training are typically anaerobic in nature. (See Anaerobic Training Effect, p. 00 and Strength Training Effects, p. 00.)

The *major organizational step* involves the

application of the elements of intensity, duration, and frequency. When strength training is first employed on a widespread basis in a particular sport, the ability of the coach to vary these three elements skillfully is not as critical as it is later. The competitive edge in simply employing a fundamentally sound strength program is proportionally greater in the first years. As time goes on and programs become more sophisticated, the importance of variation and control of the intensity, duration, and frequency in all sports will tend to increase. This has already occurred in football, the weight events in track, swimming, to some degree in college basketball, and baseball. In highly competitive situations these factors can influence winning or losing "the close ones."

The following statements are intended as guidelines to the reader. Few scientific studies offer precise answers to many of the factors involving the variation of intensity, frequency, and duration. The authors will therefore offer suggestions based upon surveys of the most successful strength programs for athletes used nationwide, as well as those developed through personal experience in the field. Wherever unbiased scientific research has illuminated a point of importance, it is documented to the readers' advantage.

Intensity

Intensity is the most important of the three elements in strength training, just as it is in aerobic and anaerobic training. In strength training the element of intensity deals with the following factors:

1. the particular exercises used,
2. the number of exercises per workout,
3. the amount of weight per set,
4. the number of sets per exercise,
5. the number of repetitions per set,
6. the time between sets, and
7. the number of repetitions per unit of time.

Intensity factor #1: The particular exercises used. In selecting the exercises to be used the purpose of each exercise must first be identified. For this reason the strength exercises have been classified into four groups according to their function, as follows:

Major exercises are those that develop the large power muscles of the body. They are explosive muscles that are used as main movers in nearly all athletic movements. The major exercises are trained with emphasis toward maximum strength. They include:

1. The Bench Press develops the large muscles of the chest, shoulders, and arms.
2. The Squat develops the muscles of the hips, thighs, and the lower back.
3. The Power Clean is a complex athletic movement that develops the muscles of the shoulders, arms, back, hips, thighs, calves, and forearms (or grip). The Power Clean should be used only when close supervision is available.

Assistant exercises are those that assist the development of maximum strength in the major exercises. The large muscles involved in the assistant exercises are the same as those involved in the major exercises. The angle of movement is changed so that the large muscle and some of the surrounding, supporting muscles are developed to a greater extent. The assistant exercises include:

1. Bar Dips assist the Bench Press.
2. Behind Neck Press assists the Bench Press.
3. Front Squat assists the Squat.
4. Incline Press assists the Bench Press.
5. Leg Press assists the Squat and Power Clean.
6. Military Press assists the Bench Press.
7. Back Squat assists the Squat.
8. Dead Lift assists the Power Clean. Some strength coaches consider the Dead Lift a major exercise. It is the authors' opinion, and the opinion of most, that the Dead Lift is an exercise that should not be trained for maximum efforts, for safety reasons. (See Dead Lift.)
9. High Pull assists the Power Clean.

Supplemental exercises are used to develop the many other muscles utilized in performing athletic movements and preventing athletic injuries. There are so many supplemental exercises that it is impractical to attempt to list them here. Among the exercises described in this chapter that are not previously listed as major or assistant exercises are the supplemental exercises. Supplemental exercises are generally designed for strength and muscular endurance. Despite this, the complex variations in repetitions, sets, and the weight used in most strength training systems are not usually applied to the supplemental exercises. Many times, supplemental exercises isolate muscle groups rather than work several or many areas as major or assistant exercises do. The supplemental exercises selected for a program vary, based on the performance needs of the sports, the special areas of injury risk presented by the sport, and the weaknesses or injury history of the individual athlete. Some supplemental exercises such as those involving the neck and, in some cases, the shoulder girdle are trained mainly for hypertrophy to prevent injuries. Others, such as leg extensions, may be used to prevent injuries by pausing or overloading in the completely extended position, thus ensuring the development of fixator muscles (those which support the knee when the foot is planted). Still other supplemental exercises such as those working on the extremities (e.g., toe raises or wrist curls) are usually trained for higher repetitions (25 to 50 or more) because of their extremely high endurance capability and utilization in the sport.

Specialty exercises are those that have been created especially for a particular sport. They are usually designed to imitate the exact range of motion used in a specific sport skill. They may, however, be designed to isolate a particular muscle group used in a sport or to strengthen one in order to help prevent an injury common to a particular sport.

The specialty exercises for each sport included in this text can be found at the end of each chapter dealing with that sport in Part II. These classifications apply directly to the free weights. Most exercise machines and other equipment can be easily adjusted to this classification system when specific exercises are not available. This can be done by substituting an assistant or a supplemental exercise to work the same area at the same intensity as the "free weight" exercise listed on the program (e.g., the Leg Press for the Squat).

Intensity factor #2: The number of exercises per workout. In determining the number of exercises to be used in each workout several criteria must be considered:

1. the time available for each workout,
2. the period in the year-round program (off-season, pre-season, or in-season),
3. the strength training equipment available,
4. the personal opinion of the athlete or coach as to which system of training best serves his needs.

In the opinion of the authors the optimal off-season strength program should involve each of the major exercises twice per week, with three or four assistant exercises done once or twice a week. This means that when the frequency of the off-season workouts is three per week, some combination of three of these exercises is contained in each workout (3 majors, or 2 majors and one assistant, or 3 assistants, etc.).

It normally requires four supplemental exercises to work on the neck, grip, calves, and abdomen in each workout. Sometimes two or more other supplemental exercises may be added to isolate areas, such as upper or lower back, knee, or ankle. These extra exercises can be alternated or rotated weekly, working them from one to three days per week. The athlete may also choose to work on one or more specialty exercises in the off-season workout, even though specialty exercises are stressed most in the pre-season and in-season.

A total of seven to twelve exercises or more can be included in the off-season program. The duration of this type of workout would be from 1½ to 2 hours or more. It is possible to shorten it to approximately an hour or less for young athletes or if time is limited. This is done by reducing the recommended number of sets, or the number of extra supplemental or specialty exercises.

The number of exercises is usually kept the same during the pre-season program, with the addition of several specialty and supplemental (injury prevention) exercises. The objective in the pre-season includes adjusting the muscular endurance to the level required in the sport. The number of exercises is therefore kept high in the pre-season to ensure the building of muscular endurance.

In season the number of exercises in each workout can usually be reduced. Concentration at this time is on injury prevention, specialty movements, and the overall maintenance of each of the major muscle groups.

Intensity factor #3: The amount of weight per set. In the off-season strength program the amount of weight per set is determined by considering the following:

1. the strength of the athlete,
2. which type of exercise is being performed (i.e., major, assistant, supplemental, or specialty),
3. the exact purpose of the set being done,
4. at what phase in the athlete's overall conditioning program the workout is to occur, and
5. the intensity level called for by the workout (light, medium, heavy, etc. See "Cycle Systems.).

A question nearly always asked by the athlete just beginning a strength program is, "What weight should I start with?" It is difficult to provide an exact answer, since the possible range of a beginner's strength is so wide. The best answer is to start with the empty bar or the lightest possible weight on the first workout, and proceed to increase the weight gradually, making sure that the proper form is maintained. After the first workout, the athlete or coach may be able to estimate or safely determine the athlete's maximum for one repetition (1RM). By knowing the "max," the starting warm-up weight can be determined by using the following table.

A guideline for increasing the amount of weight in the off-season is: "Whenever repetitions are performed, increase the weight in the next workout!" This does not apply when the athlete is involved in a "cycle system" or a program that specifically calls for less than maximum resistance levels.

Another "rule of thumb" to aid in increasing the amount of weight used is: "Always make larger, or equal, increases first." The following example will help clarify this:

Example. Assume that the athlete is performing repetition series "A"

Reps.	10	10	8	8	6	6	4	4
A Wt.	135	135	145	145	155	155	165	165
B Wt.	135	135	150	150	160	160	170	170
C Wt.	135	135	150	150	165	165	175	175

When the repetitions are accomplished and the weight is to be increased from 165 to 170, it is necessary to increase all but the first two sets. This allows that the larger (15 lb.) increase will be made first. The resulting repetition series appears as shown in series "B." The next (5 lb.) increase from 170 to 175 produces repetition series "C," which shows the first two larger (15 lb.) poundage increases first.

Starting Weight	Maximum
20–30	40–50 lbs.
35–50	55–75
55–65	80–100
70–80	105–125
85–100	130–150
105–125	155–175
135	180–Up

FIGURE 4.1 *Selection of a Starting Weight Based on 1 RM*

The first two weeks of the off-season strength program are considered the preparatory period or "preparatory phase." At this time, light-to-medium weights are used, gradually increasing into the regular off-season workout.

The off-season strength programs in this text contain the following general pattern in terms of the purpose of each set in a series. The major and assistant exercises utilize the first two sets for warm-up. Supplemental and specialty exercises require only one warm-up set. A very light weight is used for the warm-up. It must be light enough to ensure that perfect movement form is used on each repetition and that there is no thought or sign of muscular strain by the performer.

The next two or three sets are generally done with a medium amount of weight. The purpose of the medium weight is to concentrate on form and gradually adjust to the heavier amounts of weight to be handled.

The final sets of the major, assistant, and supplemental exercises are usually done with maximum weights.[15] By this is meant that the repetitions are done at the repetition maximum level where the athlete is not able to do more repetitions than the program calls for in each set. (See Repetition, p. 00)

This example shows how such a repetition series appears in the text:

Bench Press
10	10	8		8	6	6	4	4
warm-ups		medium sets			sets for 6 RM and 4 RM			

Maximum weights on the final sets can be used in nearly every workout for most off-season strength programs. The exception occurs when a cycle system is being utilized. In such cases, the program will specify the exact amount of weight to be used on a "percentage of maximum" basis.

In the pre-season and in-season strength program the amount of weight can be adjusted in a more general way. During these periods the sets are very often at the same weight. An estimate of this amount is 50 percent of 1RM, which is light enough to be used for the warm-up as well as the remaining sets. As programs and strength equipment become more specialized, the variation of the amount of weight in the pre-season and in-season will be more sophisticated. The negative performance aspects of training with too much weight in-season deter the use of wide variations in the amount of weight at this time. This is especially true in the sports activities with delicate, complex skill involvement.

Another factor which influences the overall conditioning program in-season is the intensity of the other types of conditioning. The cumulative effect of the total amount of stress and fatigue on the athlete from practice and conditioning must be carefully controlled. This may mean reducing the amount of weight used.

Intensity factor #4: The number of sets per exercise. The number of sets per exercise are determined by considering the special characteristics of the exercise itself and the seasonal point in yearly training cycle (or the "phase" of the program).

In the "preparatory phase," or the first two weeks of the off-season program, each exercise can be started with three or four sets and increased by one set per workout until the full off-season complement for each exercise is attained. In the regular off-season program, the major and assistant exercises that use large amounts of weight involve from three to five warm-up and medium weight sets before reaching the sets of maximum intensity. With the supplemental and specialty exercises, maximum resistance is usually reached after one to three sets. Then all classifications of exercises from three to five sets are usually performed at the maximum intensity level. The exception to this is the Power Clean which, although it is a major exercise, normally involves only five or six sets. These might be one warm-up, one medium, three medium heavy (done with concentration on form), and one heavy.

The major and assistant exercises are normally trained for a larger number of sets because of the fact that more adjustment intervals are necessary to reach the heavier weights. The larger muscles trained in these exercises also respond well to more sets in terms of strength development. An even larger number of heavy sets, during certain periods of the program, can be beneficial to the development of maximum strength. As sets are added, the amount of benefit derived from the addition of each successive set is gradually decreased. Therefore, the costs to the athlete in terms of the additional time and energy must be weighed against his or her personal need for additional strength.

Few sets are used in the Power Clean because of the stress created by the impact of handling a heavy weight explosively, and the need for quick-

ness and good form. Proper form and quickness decrease rapidly with fatigue.

During the pre-season and in-season strength program the number of sets per exercise usually remains constant throughout the workout. Three to five sets are recommended for the pre-season workouts and one to three sets for the in-season. This often entails a circuit training program. Exceptions to this include football linemen and linebackers who may train the upper body to develop maximum strength in season. Such workouts include Bench Presses, Incline Presses, and weighted Bar Dips. Another group of athletes who train maximally year round are the track weightmen.

The previously described tendencies represent the general pattern of sets used by the majority of collegiate and professional strength programs for athletes. The Jones System espoused by Nautilus Inc. is the major exception, employing only one or two sets of each exercise year round.

Intensity factor #5: The number of repetitions per set. The number of repetitions that should be used is determined by the immediate objective of the strength program. The ultimate objective of the program in terms of strength is to develop the greatest amount of functional strength at the endurance level of the particular sport.

Maximum strength and maximum local muscular endurance lie on opposite ends of a continuum. Each sport corresponds to a certain point on the continuum where the combination of muscular endurance versus strength is at a specific level for that activity. This may differ from position to position, even within a particular sport. If maximum muscular strength is desired, the training program will emphasize greater resistance with fewer reps. Conversely, if maximum local muscular endurance is desired, the strength program should emphasize many reps against less resistance. (See Figure 4.2). This effect is best illustrated by the work of Anderson and Kearney.[2]

Because of this continuum the athlete must train his or her muscles in season at the endurance level of the particular sport. The question is "How can one develop more force (or strength) at high endurance levels?" The answer lies in the fact that maximum strength can be developed in such large amounts at low endurance. This is done during the off-season. The transition or adjustment of this maximum strength to local muscular endurance is done during the pre-season. Because of the effect of the maximum strength versus maximum mus-

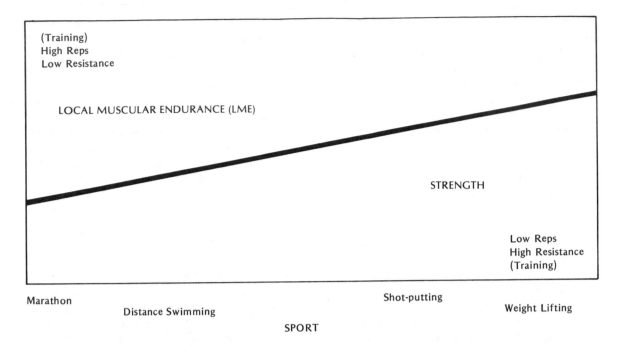

FIGURE 4.2 *Muscular Strength—Muscular Endurance Relationship*

cular endurance continuum not all of the strength will transfer. The amount that does transfer makes a significant difference in terms of functional strength at the necessary endurance level. The practical application of this fact has made strength training advantageous to athletes in nearly every sport. *More strength with endurance* can be achieved by training for maximum strength off-season, then transferring that strength to high endurance. This is much more effective in producing strength with "absolute" endurance than is training with lighter weights at high endurance year round. In this fact lies one of the key concepts in strength training for athletes.

Maximum strength is best developed by performing repetition maximums between 1RM and 8RMs. Beyond ten repetitions, increased muscular endurance becomes the dominant result. Significant strength gains have been produced at 60 percent of 1RM. Best results are achieved within the range of 80 to 100 percent of 1RM. Research directed toward this subject has shown that many variations of repetitions within the 1RM to 8RMs range are effective in producing maximum strength gains.[4, 7, 33]

Only a few exercises in an athlete's off-season program do *not* employ the one to eight "maximum strength reps." These usually include exercises for the extremities, the abdomen, and any specialty exercises involving complex movements, such as throwing or kicking. In the pre-season and in-season workouts the repetitions are adjusted as closely as is practical to the muscular endurance required by the sport.

Intensity factor #6: The time interval between sets. Controlling the time between sets is a very important part of controlling the intensity of any strength program. The criteria to be considered in varying the time intervals between sets are:

1. the amount of weight lifted,
2. the objective of the program in terms of "maximum strength versus maximum muscular endurance,"
3. the objective of the program in terms of increasing muscular size or muscular strength,
4. the importance of muscular recovery to the performance of the exercise being trained,
5. the amount of time available for the workout, and
6. the intensity of the other types of conditioning in which the athlete is involved.

When a muscle reaches momentary failure, AMF, it takes approximately five minutes for the muscle to recover 99.9 percent. Of this recovery,

95 percent occurs within 2½ minutes, 75 percent within one minute, and 50 percent within 30 seconds.[33] For this reason, athletes lifting heavy weights for maximum efforts (RMs) must rest at least two or three minutes between sets.

In the off-season major and assistant exercises are usually trained in a "set system."[11] All of the sets of one exercise are completed before beginning another exercise. When this is done, the rest intervals between sets can be gradually increased in length as the sets get heavier: 1 minute intervals after warm-up sets, 1½–2 minute intervals after medium sets, and 3–5 minute intervals after heavy sets.

If the time available for the strength workout is limited, the shorter of the suggested rest intervals can be utilized. When training an exercise that requires quickness and good form in a complex athletic movement, the athlete may benefit by using the maximum allotted time for the rest interval. The Power Clean is an example of such an exercise.

The supplemental and specialty exercises in the off-season program can employ a "circuit" system, thereby reducing the time between sets. To accomplish this, two to five exercise stations are prepared. When maximum strength is the objective, the exercises can be arranged so that consecutive exercises do not work on the same muscle groups. As a result, a rest interval of between one and 30 seconds, or less, can be achieved. The athlete can go through such a circuit by working continuously until all the sets of each exercise are completed, or can take a rest interval after one set of each exercise is completed. If a rest period is taken after each round, the time can be used to adjust the amount of weight at the various stations. In some cases the athlete may wish to develop the size and muscular definition of a certain muscle or area of the body. To do this, a bodybuilding technique, "supersets," can be used. Supersets are done by performing different exercises that continuously place stress on the same muscle group. This helps to create a better "pump" by continually forcing the blood into the muscle. The capillaries in the tissue are kept expanded for a longer period of time, the result being larger increases in muscular size. An extension of the technique used by bodybuilders is called a "blitz system."[11]

The pre-season and in-season strength programs often employ a circuit training system. In such cases the time interval between sets is usually between 3 and 10 seconds. When high intensity and the improvement of muscular endurance is desired, the athletes can run or move very quickly between stations in an attempt to get the time between sets as short as possible. If heavy weights are to be used, a "set system" is employed with the time intervals the same as those used for the major or assistant exercises in the off-season.

Intensity factor #7: The number of repetitions per unit time. As mentioned previously, opinions differ about the speed at which the strength repetitions should be performed. Information supporting fast-speed strength training was offered by Pipes and Wilmore, 1975,[35] and Counsilman.[9] Information supporting slow-speed strength training is offered by Westcott.[33] The authors have concluded that the best method is to develop strength in the off-season with heavy resistance, and then transfer the strength to fast-speed in the pre-season and in-season. With heavy weights, the intensity of the exercise does not depend as much on movement speed as it does with lighter weights.

In the pre-season and in-season the program can be rendered ineffective if the repetitions with light weights are not done at a sufficiently high speed. For example, in a pre-season or in-season circuit a station is usually designed to last for a specific time interval. This might vary from 12 seconds to one minute. If the light repetitions are performed slowly, with pauses, very little work will be performed. It is possible that some minimal amount of strength maintenance will result in this situation, but there will likely be little benefit in terms of muscular endurance. A minimum number of repetitions for each timed station should be prescribed. It is also recommended that if high intensity and high muscular endurance are desired, constant fast-speed movement should be maintained throughout the interval. This means starting the first repetition at the very beginning of the interval and not allowing the bar or the force lever of the machine to pause until the very end of the interval. Discipline and enthusiasm are required if this is to be achieved.

This method of circuit training results in an extremely high intensity level. If, as in the case of many college football programs, the pre-season entails two-a-day practices, an intense strength program of this type should be used discriminately.

Frequency

During the rest period between workouts the muscles rebuild. Waste products are eliminated from the tissues, and biochemical changes occur which cause the development of strength and/or muscular endurance. The level to which the muscle rebuilds is to a great degree dependent upon the length of the rest period and the intensity of the workout that preceded the rest period. For this reason, controlling the frequency of workouts properly has a great deal to do with the success of the strength program.

The frequency most often recommended in the off-season and pre-season is three days a week. Athletes just beginning strength training should stay on a three-day-per-week program for at least six to eight weeks, until an adjustment to the stress of strength training is made. Some athletes respond well to a regular program of four or five days per week.[35] Considering the amount of time dedicated to other areas of conditioning, it is usually advisable to wait until the second off-season program to extend beyond three days per week.

In advanced strength training programs even six- or seven-day-per-week programs are used by some individuals for limited periods of time. Programs with such high levels of stress are used to stimulate greater development by athletes who are acquainted with advanced strength training methods. To understand the value of such stressful training, it is necessary to understand the general pattern of strength development. Larger strength increases occur in the first few weeks and months of strength training. As time goes on, increases become smaller and so-called "plateaus" become longer. Some advanced individuals have found a method to help overcome such long plateaus. If the individual is in good condition, training three days a week, workouts are increased to seven days a week. This makes it impossible to recover fully between workouts. The experienced individual knows how to avoid injuries by using the proper exercises and by adjusting the weight and number of repetitions. After a number of these seven-day-per-week sessions (usually 1½ to 2½ weeks), the fatigue level has increased to the point that much lighter weights must be used. By continuing at this frequency the body gradually permits the weight to be increased again. After four to six weeks the strength level is back to the point of the original plateau. The workout frequency can then be reduced to four, five, or six days per week, depending upon how long the individual can tolerate the work level. When the days are reduced, the body is able to recover fully, developing greater strength. This method works successfully for certain individuals and in some cases has been responsible for the development of the enormous strength of the world-class weight lifters. Such high training frequencies are *definitely NOT recommended for most athletes*. Because of the success of athletes such as former world record holder and National Powerlifting Champion, John Kanter, of Phoenix, Arizona, and many others, it is not possible to discount the advantage of extremely high workout frequencies to some individuals.

The frequency of pre-season workouts is usually three days per week. When an extremely intense pre-season program or training camp is administered, two days per week is sometimes used. In these instances, the athletes are on more of a maintenance strength program rather than one geared to develop explosive strength or high muscular endurance.

The in-season strength program normally entails a frequency of one or two days per week. This is the frequency recommended by the authors. However, three-day-per-week in-season strength programs are not uncommon in some sports. There should not be a mandatory strength workout on the day prior to an athletic competition. It has been observed that some athletes prefer performing a few light sets just prior to competition. This procedure helps reduce muscle tension and partially pumps and warms up the muscles, perhaps providing some psychological as well as physical benefit. The intensity of such a warm-up should obviously be kept at a minimum.

Duration

The duration of the off-season strength workout can vary from 45 minutes to four hours. These figures, of course, represent extremely short and extremely long off-season workouts. The optimal duration for the off-season workout depends upon the relative contribution that strength training makes toward the improvement of performance in that particular sport. For example, strength training affects performance a great deal more for football linemen, or the weight events in track, than it does in cross country or golf.

The statement of this fact does not diminish the importance of strength training to success in any sport. It is rather a recognition that a higher degree of "functional strength" can be developed for certain types of athletic activities than for others. When the level of competition is so high that the margin of success is very slim, a small amount of functional strength can easily mean the difference between success and failure.

To determine the relative value of strength training versus the other types of conditioning (aerobic, anaerobic, skills, and flexibility training), a concept dealing with the economic use of time is necessary. A law of economics called "The Law of Diminishing Return" needs to be considered in this situation. This law states that when an investment is made in a productive area, a return results; however, as continuing investments in the same area are made, the return becomes progressively smaller.

In the case of strength training for a football lineman the return on the investment of time does not diminish as rapidly as it does for a complex skill activity such as golf. The first hour and a half of investment for the football lineman and for the golfer yield a great return in terms of improved performance. When a golfer's workout is extended beyond an hour and a half, the amount of beneficial return is reduced considerably. At this point it becomes more likely that the extra time would have been better spent on skills training. If the workouts were extended to 2½ or 3 hours, it is almost a certainty that an extra hour of practicing golf would have been a wiser use of the available time. The same cannot be said for the football lineman, since the strength training done during the third and even the fourth hours of his workout might benefit him more than extra hours of addi-

tional skills practice. The relative value of increasing the duration of the workout, in terms of the improved performance of the individual athlete, must be carefully considered when planning workouts.

At the junior high and high school levels there is often a "class period" limitation of the amount of time available for off-season strength training. In such situations the workout must be compressed. This can be done by: 1) shortening the time between sets, 2) training the major exercises in a circuit, or 3) training five or six days per week on a "split routine" (upper body one day, lower body the next).

During the pre-season and in-season the duration of the workouts is greatly reduced. For most sports a 20-30 minute circuit can be employed effectively in the pre-season. The duration of an in-season workout is even shorter, usually ranging from 7 to 15 minutes. If a heavy workout is to be used during this period by a special group or individual such as a football lineman, an additional 20-30 minutes should be allowed.

Devising Strength Programs

Any strength program for athletes that follows the principles, essentials, and elements previously described in this chapter should produce significant strength gains. As mentioned previously, large in-

	Off-Season	Pre-Season	In-Season
INTENSITY			
Amount of Resistance	Heavy	Light	Lighter
Speed of Exercises	Slow	Fast	Faster
Total Number of Exercises	7 to 12	8 to 12	7 to 10
Number of Major Exercises	2-3	2-3	2-3
Sets	8-10	5	2-3
Reps	1-8	10-50	10-50
Number of Assistant Exercises	1-2	1-2	1-2
Sets	6-8	5	2-3
Reps	1-8	10-50	10-50
Number of Supplemental Exercises	3-5	3-5	3-5
Sets	3-5	5	2-5
Sets	3-5	5	2-3
Reps	8-30	10-50	10-50
Number of Specialty Exercises	1-3	1-3	1-3
Sets	3-5	5	2-3
Reps	10-50	10-50	10-50
FREQUENCY			
Days/Week	3-5	3	1-2
DURATION			
Workout Time	45 min.-4 hrs.	20-30 min.	7-15 min.

FIGURE 4.3 *The Year-Round Variance of the Elements of Intensity, Frequency, and Duration.*

creases in strength will occur within the first six to eight weeks. Later the gains are smaller and generally occur more slowly. The tendency toward slower and smaller strength increases must be recognized and accepted. In the view of the authors, the existence of actual strength "plateaus" is questionable. The reason for the concept of the "strength plateau" is that in most cases the athlete has considered his strength based solely upon his 1RM. As was pointed out in the discussion concerning "number of repetitions," training with repetitions between 1RM and 8RMs produces strength increases that are not significantly different. Since the goal of the athlete is not the increase of the 1RM alone, the suggestion is made that within the range of 1RM to 8RMs, strength improvements can be occurring constantly. In order for this to occur, the athlete must know how to utilize the correct strength system.

The effectiveness of various types of strength training programs has been studied in recent years. Berger, DeLorme, and Watkins did classic early studies in this area. Numerous other persons have also contributed substantial research in this area.[35] Beyond the basic indications that heavy low repetitions (1–8 RM) are most effective in producing maximum strength gains, no repetition series or pattern of progressively increasing resistance has been found to be clearly superior. Most strength experts readily agree that the method that works best for one individual may not at all be best for another. In fact, the best program for an individual during a particular off-season may not be the best for the same individual the next off-season.

Figure 4.4 shows some commonly used repetition series with the resistance levels or increases indicated by the "step-like" lines.

A method of increasing strength while main-

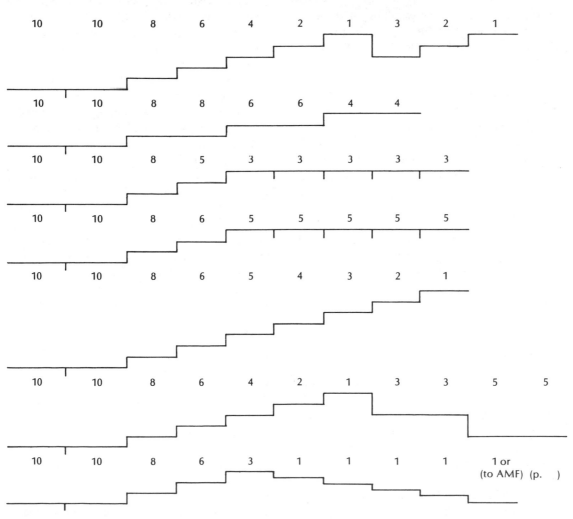

FIGURE 4.4 *Repetition Series for Major and Assistant Exercises*

taining a repetition level that can be increased is as follows:

In one workout on a major or assistant exercise, the athlete finds his or her RM for two repetition levels (example 3RM and 5RM). In the next Monday workout the athlete performs the following repetition series:

| 10 | 10 | 8 | 5 | 3 | 3 | 3 | 3 | 3 |

The 3s are done at a resistance level of 3 RM minus 10 pounds. If three sets of three reps are performed successfully, the five sets of three reps are increased in the following Monday workout. The increase should be +5 pounds for upper body exercises and +10 pounds for lower body exercises. Do not exceed this amount of increase. If three sets of three repetitions are not performed successfully, the weight remains the same the following week. If at any time the repetitions are not performed successfully for three consecutive weeks, the weight is increased by the called-for amount (+5 or +10 pounds) and the repetitions are changed to 2s. The following repetition series results:

| 10 | 8 | 6 | 4 | 2 | 2 | 2 | 2 | 2 |

On Friday this same procedure is used with five repetitions at 5RM (10 pounds): 10, 10, 8, 6, 5, 5, 5, 5, 5. Again, three sets must be performed successfully in order to increase the resistance the following week. When this cannot be achieved for three weeks, the 5s are increased in weight and become 4s: 10, 10, 8, 6, 4, 4, 4, 4, 4.

This procedure can be continued until the reps become 1s. The program series on that day can then be started again with 8s, as follows:

| 10 | 10 | 8 | 8 | 8 | 8 | 8 | 8 |

Cycle Systems

Cycle systems were developed to help avoid overtraining, eliminate guesswork, and ensure that "peaking out" occurs at the proper time. When strength programs are extended continuously throughout the months of the off-season, overtraining becomes a definite problem. The cycle programs allow for the necessary "recovery" as well as "overload." In junior high school and college level sports in the United States this type of program is not usually necessary. This is because the athlete's off-season strength program normally extends for only six to a maximum of ten weeks, after which a lengthy interruption occurs. When an athlete's strength program extends beyond ten weeks, including the two-week preparatory period, a cycle program of some type should be employed.

The sports situations in the United States in which cycle systems are most commonly used are in the weight events in track, where heavy strength training occurs throughout the in-season period, and in professional sports, where uninterrupted training occurs throughout the off-season. In college football—which would otherwise lend itself well to cycle programs—the placement of spring football permits only a six- to ten-week off-season strength program. These problems, along with others such as multiple sport high school situations, limit the effectiveness and therefore the application of cycle systems in this country.

Cycle systems are constructed using several different guidelines to adjust the amount of weight, the number of repetitions, and the spacing of the recovery period. Cycle systems are characterized by the utilization of a recovery (or light) week every three or four weeks. The amount of weight or the overall intensity of the program handled each week is varied. The training week is rated as follows: 1) heavy, 2) medium heavy, 3) medium, or 4) light. The individual workout intensity may also be rated in the same way.

In some cases the workout rating system is based upon the number of repetitions performed within a certain percentage (e.g., 50 percent) of the athlete's 1RM. This would include only repetitions done in the major or assistant exercises. Another method used in this text to present a cycle program for track weight events utilizes the percentage of a projected 1RM to rate the weekly and daily workouts. The details of this system are presented in Chapter 16. This program can easily be adapted to strength programs for any sport if extended off-season periods are available. To accomplish this, substitute the described cycle system into the major and assistant exercises recommended in the off-season program for the appropriate sport.

Safety Procedure

Weight training can be one of the safest of physical activities. The authors, however, must caution the novice to seek help from a coach or knowledgeable weight trainer *before attempting* unfamiliar lifts. It is wise even for athletes with some experience at weight training to have new exercises explained or demonstrated. Most of the injuries that occur are muscle and tendon strains.

It seems likely that weight-lifting strains might aggravate or even cause hernia injuries, but such injuries are rare among weight lifters. It is safe to assume that most injuries incurred in weight training could have been prevented by the application of common sense and a few safety techniques.

1. The *weight belt* should be used when doing any moderately heavy or heavy weight training. The belt helps to prevent back and abdominal injuries. A competition belt is a maximum of four inches wide. An athlete, however, can use an even wider belt while training for sports.
2. Check the equipment you are using *before performing each exercise.*
   a. Collars on the bar need to be tight. Sometimes the threads will become stripped and although the collar may appear to be tight, if the bar is tilted it will slip off.
   b. Check the condition of cables and pulleys on all equipment. Worn-out or partially worn-through cables and ropes should not be used.
   c. All bolts and screws on Olympic bars or other equipment and machines should be checked for tightness.
3. It is best to have *two spotters* available during weight training sessions. The spotters are particularly necessary when performing the Bench Press, the Squat, and the Incline Press. Other exercises, such as Supine Tricep Extensions, Seated Press Behind the Neck, and Lat Pulls, can also require spotters.
4. *Good lifting technique* is one of the most important ways of preventing back injuries. When lifting any weight and particularly a heavy weight from the ground, the knees should be bent and the back should be kept straight with the head up. There are some exercises, such as Toe Touches and the Good Morning exercise, which are done by bending at the waist with the knees straight. These exercises are the exception to the bent leg rule, but only light weights are used.

DESCRIPTIONS OF STRENGTH EXERCISES

The following are explanations of how to do the various exercises that will be used in the strength programs in this book. The exercises are provided in more or less alphabetical order so that you may refer to them easily. In order to understand the exercise descriptions and programs that follow, several terms that will be used to describe body movements need to be defined.

Flexion and *Extension*. When discussing joint flexion, the decreasing angle of the joint is used to indicate that the joint is being flexed. An increasing joint angle therefore indicates joint extension. A muscle is *flexed* when it is contracted, making it shorter. For example, in the Bench Press contraction of the tricep muscles causes extension of the elbow joints. Therefore, unless otherwise designated, flexion and extension will refer to joint flexion and joint extension.

Prone and *Supine*. The supine position is lying on the back face up. Prone is the opposite—lying on the stomach, face down.

Bar Dips

This exercise is done on parallel bars. The player mounts the bar in a straight-arm support position with the elbows extended, then lowers position until the middle of the chest is even with the bars. Flexing the elbows, the athlete then drives explosively back to the starting position. Repeat this pattern. After working up to ten reps for five sets, the athlete is ready to use weights for the dip. Bar Dips develop the chest, shoulders, and arms. The bottom part of the pectoralis is affected more strongly. Training with this exercise may be helpful in preventing many shoulder injuries.

Behind Neck Press

Just as the name describes, presses are done by lowering the bar behind the neck. The bar is either taken from a rack, at shoulder level, or handed to the athlete with the arms held straight upward and the elbows extended. The movement is then performed by lowering the bar behind the head to a level below the ears and driving it back overhead.

PHOTO 4.1   *Bar Dips*

For the full range of motion, the bar is brought down to touch the very base of the neck. Some individuals, however, find this puts excess strain on the posterior head of the deltoids and/or the insertions of the trapezius muscles. It is acceptable to begin slowly in gaining the full range of motion in this exercise, or if necessary, only to lower the bar to a level that is even with the ears.

Bench Press

This exercise is done in the supine position. The athlete should grip the bar with the hands, approxi-mately at shoulder width, evenly spaced from the middle of the bar. Spotters are recommended to aid in getting the bar off the rack and into position. The bar is then lowered straight to the chest. There is a range of several inches in the position of the bar on the chest. The best position is usually at the origin of the pectoralis major or about six to eight inches below the shoulder sockets. From there the bar is moved to a position directly above the shoulders. The bar should be driven to that position in a straight line.

This exercise is an excellent one to develop the large muscles of the chest, shoulders, and arms—pectoralis major and minor, deltoids, and

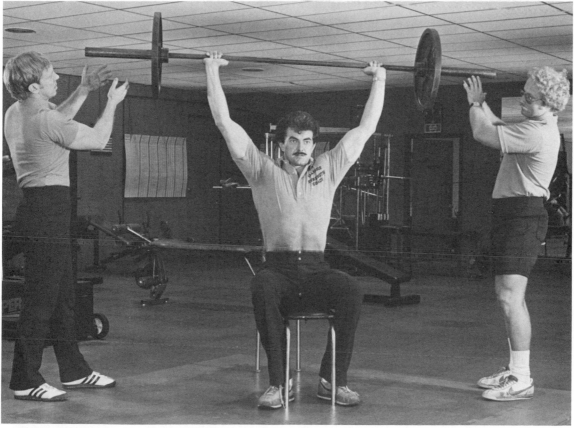

PHOTO 4.2 *Behind Neck Press*

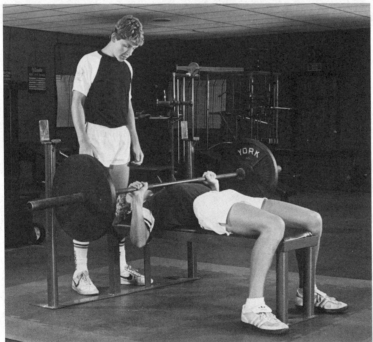

PHOTO 4.3   *Bench Press*

triceps. The strength of these muscles will determine the individual's explosive power in the upper body. These muscles are the main movers for most athletic movements, so it is not difficult to realize why the Bench Press is used for strength development in nearly every sport. (The exclusion of any one of these three main muscle groups will limit the performance of most athletic movements.)

Bent Arm Laterals (or Fly)

This exercise is done in the supine position (preferably on a bench), using a dumbbell in each hand. Begin with the dumbbells directly above the shoulder sockets, with the elbows slightly flexed and the hands held palms in. The elbows remain flexed throughout the movement. They are laterally lowered until the dumbbells are even with the sides—then back above the shoulders again.

Bent Arm Pullovers

This exercise is also done in the supine position on a bench or with the head and upper shoulders supported on a bench. The exercise is usually done with a dumbbell but can be done by using an easy curl bar or a close grip on a barbell. The weight is held directly above the shoulders with the elbows slightly bent (flexed). It is then lowered behind the head toward the floor, with the elbows kept

PHOTO 4.4 *Bent Arm Laterals*

PHOTO 4.5   *Bent Arm Pullovers*

flexed in this position. The extreme position of the range of motion has the upper arms even with the ears. The muscles of the lower chest are completely extended in this position. The weight is then brought back to the starting position by contracting the muscles of the lower chest and abdomen. During the entire movement the elbows are kept in so that they pass close to the head. With a dumbbell (especially a large one) the elbows are not flexed as much in the starting position (Picture A). With a barbell or curling bar, the flexing of the elbow is even greater, since the bar is held at the chest in the starting position (Picture B). If the elbows are extended in the starting position, the triceps or elbow extensor muscles are exercised more. By bringing the bar directly to the chest, the lower chest and abdomen muscles are exercised more and the triceps less. If heavy weight is to be used, spotters may be necessary. The throwing pullover is another variation of the pullover—designed to help develop throwing velocity. (See *Throwing*.)

Bent Over Rowing

This is done by bending forward at the waist until the upper body is parallel to the floor. Either a barbell or two dumbbells are held in the hands. The arms are held downward directly toward the floor. If a padded, waist-high head support is available, it is advantageous to support the head to prevent movement of the trunk. The forehead, then, is placed on the head support. The movement is done by flexing the elbows and pulling the weight to the chest. The dumbbells may be pulled a little farther than the bar. Thus a fuller range of movement is one advantage of using dumbbells for this exercise.

Power Clean

In the Clean the barbell is brought from the floor to the chest in one continuous movement. The starting position is extremely important. The head is kept up, with the eyes focused at a point straight ahead. The bar is gripped at approximately shoulder width, with the elbows extended straight down to the bar. The feet are positioned with the heels from nine to fourteen inches apart, and the middle of the foot directly below the bar. The toes can be pointed straight ahead or slightly outward. The knees are kept inside the arms, and it is most important that the back be kept straight.

As the beginning or *drive* phase of the movement is started, the legs and hips are used to pull the bar from the floor. The athlete should concentrate on driving with the legs and thrusting the head straight toward the ceiling. In this way the back and arms are kept perfectly straight. The arms are not bent (or flexed) until the body is completely extended. The drive phase should be done explosively so that the bar is accelerating through this part of the movement. Then, as the elbows begin to flex, the body is beginning to move downward. Notice at this time that the knees are flexed as much as necessary to get the shoulders under the bar. The elbows are not passively flexing at this time, but are continuing to accelerate the bar straight up with a quick ripping movement.

PHOTO 4.6 *Bent Over Rowing*

Throughout this movement the body is very close to the bar. As the athlete drops quickly under the bar, the elbows are thrust forward and the bar comes to rest high on the chest and shoulders. Notice at this point that the back is again straight, even though the knees are flexed. The Clean is completed when the athlete brings the bar from the squatting position and stands erect with it.

PHOTO 4.7 *Power Clean*

Squat Clean

This method of cleaning a barbell is used by most Olympic-style weight lifters. It is very similar to the Power Clean. In fact, the movement is identical for the lifter during the power phase, until he or she begins to drop under the weight. At that point, in the Squat Clean the lifter begins to move the body under the weight. As the weight contacts the shoulders, the momentum of the weight is allowed to drive the legs out of the Power Clean position into the squatting position. If this is to be done successfully, the proper balance between the lifter and the weight must be maintained throughout the movement.

Split Clean

This is another effective and more traditional way of cleaning a weight to the shoulders in one move-

ment. In this movement, after the power phase the athlete drops to a split position below the weight. This is done by thrusting one leg straight backward and the other leg slightly forward—dropping to a flexed position. The back leg is kept extended nearly completely through the knee joint. The same leg is usually used for each repetition, but alternating the legs can be done if desired.

Curl

The Curl can be done in many different ways. It is simply the flexing of the elbow against a resistance held in the hands or hand, with the palms facing forward (anatomical position).

The Curl is distinguished from other movements involving flexion of the elbows by the fact that "flexors of the elbow" are the only muscles involved in the movement. The regular standing Curl is done by first grasping the bar at approxi-

PHOTO 4.8 *Curl*

mately shoulder width grip and lifting the bar to
the starting, standing position with the arms down
at the sides. The elbows are flexed, bringing the
weight as close to the shoulders as possible. The
feet are also approximately shoulder width apart
and the body is kept rigid throughout the movement. Complete flexion and extension are desirable in the Curl if flexibility for athletics is the
desired result.

Cable Curl

This can be done if wall pulleys are present. It can
be done from a standing position or a sitting position. From the sitting position, however, the exercise is not a true Curl but is similar to Bent Over
Rowing since the muscles of the upper back are
main movers.

PHOTO 4.9 *Cable Curl*

Close Grip Curls

These are simply regular standing Curls done with the hands held at close grip. The close grip causes greater isolation of the biceps, brachiolis, and brachioradialis, thus helping to strengthen this area.

Reverse Curl

This is done by reversing the grip on the bar so that the palms face downward instead of forward. This isolates the brachioradialis, which is one of the strongest muscles of the forearm. The movement should be done with the elbows kept close to the body and the wrists as straight as possible.

Support Curl (or Scott Curl)

This curl is done by stabilizing the elbow on a pad or brace, so that the flexors of the elbows are iso-

PHOTO 4.10 *Reverse Curl*

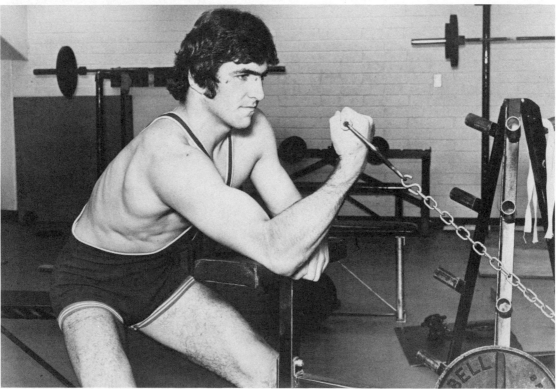

PHOTO 4.11 *Support Curl*

lated. Cable Curls or Reverse Curls may be done in this way as well when great isolation of the biceps is desired.

Dead Lift

The Dead Lift is an exercise designed to develop the powerful muscles of the thighs, hips, and lower back, which are critical in most athletic movements.

The athlete grasps a barbell and moves it from the floor to a position where he or she is standing upright, with the elbows extended straight downward supporting the weight. It is extremely important that this movement be done properly because of the hip and back stresses that can be experienced when handling a heavy weight.

The starting position is exactly the same as in the Clean, except in some cases one of the hands is reversed to provide a better grip for heavy weight. The head is kept up with the eyes focused at a point straight ahead. The bar is gripped at approximately shoulder width, with the elbows extended straight down to the bar. The feet are positioned with the heels from nine to fourteen inches apart and the middle of the foot is directly below the bar. The toes can be pointed straight ahead or slightly outward. The knees are kept inside the arms and *it is most important that the back be kept straight.*

As the movement is started, the legs and hips are used to pull the bar from the floor. The athlete should concentrate on driving with the legs and thrusting the head straight toward the ceiling. In this way the back and arms are kept perfectly straight throughout the movement. As the bar is raised the hips are moving forward until the body is straight and the Dead Lift is complete.

Dumbbell Exercises

Dumbbells are used for many movements in order to get greater isolation of a particular muscle or muscle group. They are also used to allow greater

PHOTO 4.12 *Dead Lift*

(a)

(b)

(c)

PHOTO 4.13   *Dumbbell Exercises. Dumbbell Incline Press* freedom of movement in many cases, for example, when rotation of the shoulder is desired and is not possible with a bar (Picture A). Dumbbells also have the advantage of allowing a "true" full range of motion in some exercises such as the Bench Press (Picture B) and the Incline Press (Picture C).

"Good Mornings"

This exercise is begun by grasping a light barbell at slightly wider than shoulder width grip and placing it on the shoulders behind the head. It is best to have "squat racks" on which to set the weight. If they are not available, the bar must be cleaned and pressed overhead, then lowered to the shoulders. The bar will usually rest most comfortably just above the scapula bones. Keeping the head up and the back straight (Picture A), the movement is then performed by bending forward at the waist, keeping the knees nearly extended, until the upper torso is parallel to the ground, and then going back to the starting position. As heavier weights are used, the knees must be flexed slightly to compensate the weight enough so that the center of gravity stays above the feet.

Grip Exercises

The development of the Grip requires the training of thumb and finger flexors as well as forearm flexors and extensors. Development of strength in this area many times requires extremely persistent efforts.

In training for the Grip, many different tools and methods are effective. (For example: a rubber ball or hand gripper, spring devices, wrist roller, objects carried with the thumb and fingers extended downward.) In the illustration two weights are held together with the finger and thumb joints extended downward.

Wrist Curl or Forearm Curl

This exercise is done by grasping a light barbell at shoulder width grip and supporting the forearms on a flat surface with the palms upward. The finger joints are flexed and extended throughout the full range of motion, allowing the bar to roll down the fingers as far as possible, then brought back into the fist again. This develops the flexors of the wrist.

(a)

(b)

PHOTO 4.14 *"Good Mornings"*

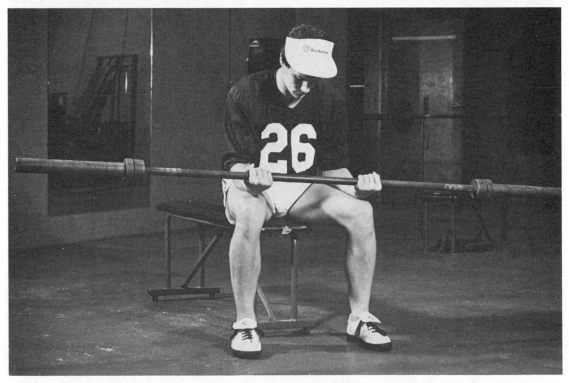

PHOTO 4.15 *Wrists Curls*

Reverse Forearm Curl

This is done in a similar manner by simply changing the grip so that the palms face downward. The exercise is more difficult this way and a lighter weight may be needed. The extensors of the wrists are the benefited muscles.

High Pull

The starting position and power phase of the High Pull are identical to those of the Power Clean. (See *Power Clean*.)

It should be remembered that these are powerful athletic movements and require sophisticated

PHOTO 4.16 *High Pull*

muscular control to be done properly. For many people, time is required to learn the basic form. It can occur almost automatically or can take several weeks. For safe execution, this basic form must be learned with very light weights—before weights requiring forceful efforts are used.

As the movement is being learned the amount of weight can be increased after two or three sessions—as long as the correct form is being used.

Snatch Pull

This exercise is another type of High Pull in which the bar is held with a very wide grip. The pull is slightly different and, consequently, the effect on the body is different. Greater development is offered in the shoulders and upper back. The timing of the explosive part of the movement is slightly quicker and lower than in the High Pull or the Clean Pull. The wider grip also creates greater stress on the hands. The increased difficulty in gripping the bar can be decreased, for training purposes, by using pull straps to help the grip so that the other muscles can be worked thoroughly.

Hyperextension

The Hyperextension gets its name from the hyperextension of the back that occurs at the top of the power phase of the movement. The hips and legs are supported so that the upper torso can bend forward to become perpendicular to the floor (Picture A). The hands are held behind the head with the fingers interlocked. From here the movement is done by contracting the muscles of the hips and of the lower back, moving the upper body to a completely extended position—somewhat greater than 180 degrees.

In training for the Hyperextension, a weight may be held behind the head. In order to prevent possible injury, it is wise to do the exercise with no weight at all for at least one or two exercise sessions. This is especially true if this exercise is being done for the very first time.

Leg Curl

The Leg Curl is usually done in the prone position on a leg extension or leg curl machine (Picture A, page 66). The knee or knees are taken from the fully

PHOTO 4.17   *Snatch Pull*

(a)

(b)

PHOTO 4.18 *Hyperextension*

PHOTO 4.19   *Incline Press*

PHOTO 4.20 *Lat Pulls*

extended position to a point where the knee joint is flexed ninety degrees or more. It can be done by using ankle weights or a weighted boot. Some training devices allow the Leg Curl to be done in the sitting position.

The affected area in the Leg Curl can be altered by changing the angle of the foot on the resistance arm of the machine.

Leg Press

In this exercise the knee goes from a flexed to an extended position, while the back remains somewhat stabilized. There are several types of leg presses, in nearly all directions.

The Leg Press is an assistant exercise to help develop hip and leg strength. Hamstrings and lower abdomen are also developed by some leg presses. The effects of different "leg press" equipment vary. The Leg Press is beneficial, however, in some situations because of its restrictive nature. An improper angle of body support and exceedingly high internal pressures can be experienced,

causing damage to joints such as knees, hips, and the spinal column. *Proceed gradually and use care and common sense when attempting extremely heavy leg presses.*

Military Press

This exercise is done by simply standing straight with a barbell supported on the hands and shoulders and pressing it straight overhead. In this movement the body should be kept as straight as possible and the knees should not bend. The Military Press develops the upper arms (triceps), the shoulders (deltoids and trapezius), and the upper chest.

To execute the Military Press, the barbell may be cleaned to the shoulders or taken from a rack, then driven explosively upward until the elbows are extended. The press rack would be most preferable for someone who wanted to concentrate on pressing in particular. In many cases, the Clean is trained separately from the Press, since maximum strength in most cases is not necessary during any one workout.

(a)

(b)

PHOTO 4.21   *Leg Curl*

PHOTO 4.22 *Military Press*

Neck Exercises

The neck is capable of several types of movement, such as: raising of the shoulders (shrugging—discussed under *Shoulder Shrug*); flexion (lowering the head toward the chest); extension (raising the head, or the opposite of flexion); lateral flexion (lowering the head toward the shoulder on either side), and rotation (moving the head on the vertical axis in both directions, as if shaking the head to say "No").

The flexion and extension movements can be done with a standard neck harness, a wrestler's bridge, or in other ways. The flexion movement is usually not as strong as extension with the standard neck harness. The weight is hung behind the head at about the middle of the back. The neck is extended as far as possible in the starting position, and then the movement is flexed as far as possible. With a neck device such as that employed on the Universal Gym or the Nautilus Neck Machine, greater resistance is provided throughout the full range of motion. (See *Nautilus Four-way Direct Neck Machine* in Appendix.)

Neck flexion is many times the only trained exercise using the neck harness. If the weight is to be hung from the harness, a stabilizing position of the upper body is important. This position can be done by placing the hands on the knees and keeping the back straight in either the sitting or standing position (Pictures A and B).

Lateral flexion is done on either the Universal neck device or the Nautilus Neck Machine. (See *Nautilus Four-way Direct Neck Machine* in Appendix.)

Neck Rotation

At this time, neck rotation muscles must be developed by hand resistance or by a special machine such as the Nautilus Rotary Neck Machine. (See Appendix.)

Power Back

This piece of equipment (Picture A) has removable pins so that the weight can be lifted off at many different heights. This allows several different

(a)

(b)

PHOTO 4.23 *Neck Flexion*

exercises to be trained on it, with many different starting levels in any one movement. The Power Rack is many times called an Isometric-Isotonic Power Rack. When pins are placed above the bar and the athlete attempts to move the bar past the pins, isometric contractions are possible. By placing weight on the bar it is possible to create a minimum force level throughout an isometric contraction.

Rack Bench

The bench is set under the power rack. The pins are set at the desired height above the athlete's chest as he or she lies on the bench. Nine to twelve inches is usually a good height. The bar is placed on the pins, then the weight is loaded. The athlete is positioned on the bench beneath the weight in the Bench Press position. From here the bar is driven off the pins, extending the elbows through the partial Bench Press movement.

The Rack Bench is done to increase tricep and deltoid power. A greater pressure than a person might be accustomed to can be placed upon the deltoids.

Rack Press

The Rack Press can be done from shoulder height, but it is considered to be a partial press off a high rack. The deltoid, trapezoid, and tricep muscles are developed. A weight belt should be used for this exercise. After the desired height has been selected and the bar is in position and loaded, the movement is done by standing directly under the bar, gripping it at approximately shoulder width, and pressing it overhead.

Rack Squat

This exercise is done to develop the hips, thighs, and back above the level that is possible with the regular Squat. To execute the movement, the back should be kept straight and the head up. Although the movement encompasses almost the same distance as the one-quarter or one-half Squat, the Rack Squat is better for developing maximum strength for several reasons. The weight is stationary, and therefore inertia must be overcome to move the weight, making starting to move the weight difficult. This factor encourages the development of explosiveness. The bar is supported so

that it can be attacked at the most difficult point—whenever the athlete is ready. From the safety standpoint, the weight cannot get outside the rack or go below the starting position. If the athlete cannot complete the movement, the bar is simply lowered to the pins, thereby relieving the athlete of the weight.

For most training purposes, the bar for the Rack Squat can be set at waist level.

Rack Dead Lift

This exercise is done to improve the Dead Lift power. Most athletes do not require heavy work on the Dead Lift or Rack Dead Lift, as it can be quite exhausting to the hips and lower back. The Rack Dead Lift has the same advantages over the regular Dead Lift as the Rack Squat has over the Squat. More weight can usually be handled through the movement than in the Dead Lift. The bar is confined within the rack, and the grip is also strengthened and confidence in handling heavy weight increased.

The Rack Dead Lift strengthens the same muscle groups as the Dead Lift. Like the Dead Lift, it can be trained for maximum efforts only over limited periods before rests are necessary.

Pulldowns

The Pulldown is done to strengthen the muscles of the lower chest and back. Using the "lat machine," the athlete either sits or kneels (just as in the Lat Pull) and the bar is pulled down in front of the body. Either a close grip or a shoulder width grip can be used. The close grip puts a greater stress on the wrists and forearms. The movement is similar to the Pullover, but the resistance is applied at a different angle.

Pull Straps

The use of pull straps will aid the grip when the bar or dumbbell is to be pulled up from the floor and/or held with the weight supported by the grip alone.

This technique should be used only to aid the grip so that other muscles can be worked thoroughly. Many times the grip fatigues before the "main mover." It is for this reason that pull straps are used. When the grip alone can do the job, it should be utilized.

When two pull straps are necessary, cotton, nylon, or leather straps are usually used. They should be from sixteen to twenty inches long and approximately one inch wide. The straps are held by wrapping them around the wrists and through the hands. It helps to keep the ends even.

If the athlete is right-handed, the left strap is wrapped first. The strap is then wrapped under the bar and the wrist is pulled down tight against the bar. The strap is then pulled around the bar next to the thumb, and is held in place by the thumb, palm, and fingers. The other hand is then wrapped; this is a little more difficult to do because the strap must be held by the fingers of the same hand to pull the wrist down to the bar and complete the wrap.

Shoulder Shrugs

These are used to develop the trapezius muscles, which serve to elevate the shoulders.

In the standing position the bar is held in the hands, with the arms suspended straight down from the shoulders (Picture A). The movement is performed by shrugging the shoulders, i.e., pulling them up toward the ears.

This may be done by pulling the shoulders straight up for a moment, then straight back down (Picture A), or by rolling the shoulders in either direction. When the movement is developed, pull straps or straps with hooks may be used.

Sit-Ups

These are done to develop the abdominal muscles. Many variations of Sit-ups can be done. For regular Sit-ups the knees should be kept flexed, relieving undesirable stress on the lower back. The hands may be held behind the head, down at the sides, crossed over the chest, or used to hold a weight on the chest (Picture A). It is best for the feet to be held down by a partner if a Sit-up board is not available. As the movement is done, the trunk may be rotated or twisted to help maintain trunk flexibility and also to aid the development of the throwing movement, which utilizes the diagonal twisting movement of the trunk. Resistance is added by holding a weight flat on the chest.

(a)

(b)

PHOTO 4.24   *Shoulder Shrugs*

Speed Exercises

A series of exercises used by sprinters to increase their running speed are discussed below. Athletes from many sports can benefit from the development of running speed, particularly in the use of the quick start.

Leg Curl for Speed

The Leg Curl is done in the prone position on the leg curl device. The toes are kept together, with the heels apart on the pads of the machine. This

(a)

(b)

PHOTO 4.25 *Sit-ups*

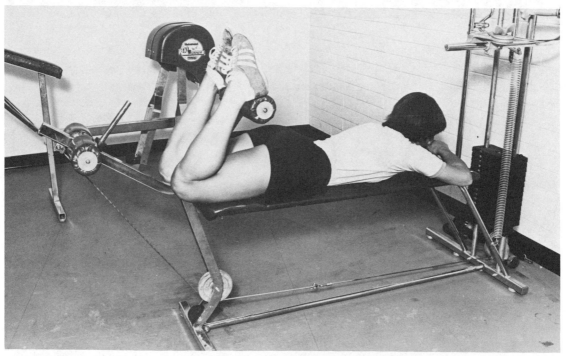

PHOTO 4.26 *Leg Curl for Speed*

foot angle tends to isolate the long flexor muscle or semitendinosus. The hips should remain flat and against the bench so that the muscle gets complete extension. At the end of the movement the knee should be flexed well past ninety degrees for most individuals. The foot position causes knee flexion to be restricted slightly. Only light weights, generally from ten to thirty pounds, are used. Light stretching, in the sprinter's position, should follow this exercise.

High Knee Lift

This exercise is done by many sprinters in order to give them more power through the drive position (Picture A)—or, as some would say, "I get better knee lift." The exercise can be done in several different ways. One way is to allow a weight to rest on the thigh near the knee, holding it there for a timed interval (Picture A). A pulley can also be attached below (Pictures B and C) or behind the runner. This exercise should be worked explosively, if possible, and high speed equipment should be used if it is available.

Leg Drive

This exercise helps the runner get a quicker start from the sprinter (Picture A) or "DOWN" (Picture B) position. A Universal Gym Leg Press Station or a Marcy Gym Leg Drive can be used. The exercise is done one leg at a time, with the same shoulder being supported as that which is driving. The athlete should keep his or her head up to imitate the running position. The foot is placed firmly upon the center of the pedal. It is best for the knee

(a)

(b)

(c)

PHOTO 4.27 *High Knee Lift*

PHOTO 4.28   *Leg Drive*

to be placed at an angle greater than ninety degrees at the start. The leg and hip drive backward explosively, obtaining complete extension of the hip and knee. The explosive movement cannot be done smoothly on some Universal Gyms and must be done at a slower speed.

Squat

The Squat is probably the best exercise for the development of the legs and hips. The back erector

muscles are also strengthened. A weight belt should be used when doing the Squat with weights. The Squat can be done to various depths. To specify which of these movements is which, they are called Quarter Squat, Half Squat, Full Squat, and Deep Squat (Pictures A–D).

When first starting to train with this exercise, light weights are used and Full Squats or Deep Squats are not done. *Persons under sixteen years of age should never do Full Squats with heavy weights.*

To perform the Squat, the bar is placed on a rack just below shoulder height. The athlete posi-

(a) *Position of Bar*

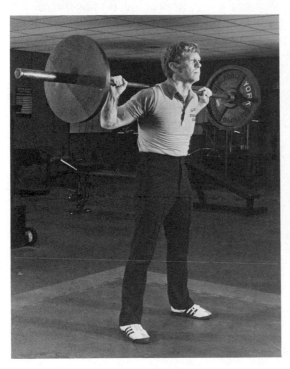

(b) *Starting and Finishing Position*

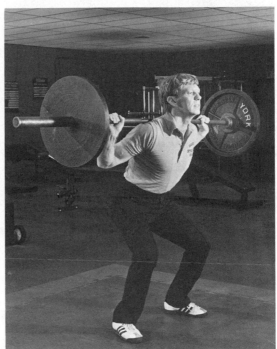

(c) *¼ Squat*

PHOTO 4.29   *Squat*

tions the bar on the back just above the scapula, on the trapezius muscle (Picture A) and takes it from the rack. *The back is kept straight in the Squat by keeping the chest out and the head up at all times* while handling the weight—both while removing it from the rack and while performing the movement. To help ensure that this position is maintained, a spot can be placed on the ceiling approximately one foot in front of the point directly above the squatter's head. *The athlete should* then *keep the eyes focused on the spot throughout the entire movement.* The weight is

removed from the rack by extending the knees and taking the weight onto the back. The athlete then takes one step backward to be in position to squat the weight. *The feet are placed at shoulder width or wider*, with the toes pointed slightly outward (Picture B).

From there, the Squat is performed by flexing the knees and hips until the thighs, or at least the bottom of the thighs, are parallel to the floor. To get the maximum benefit from the Squat, *the athlete must be sure to squat low enough.* The major effort is made as the knees and hips are extended,

(d) *½ Squat*

(e) *Full Squat*

(f) *Deep Knee Bend*

PHOTO 4.29   *Squat (Continued)*

raising the bar to the starting position. The athlete should begin the upward movement by concentrating first on extending the hips. When this is done correctly, *the hips seem to roll forward slightly under the bar* as it is raised, so that the back stays as erect as possible. This causes the final part of the upward movement to be, for the most part, knee extension.

Some athletes may prefer to use knee wraps when squatting—especially when Full Squats are to be done.

Stiff-legged Dead Lift (Caution: Use light weight.)

This exercise strengths the lower back and hamstrings. The movement is similar to the "Good Mornings." The difference in the two exercises is that the weight is held in the hands instead of upon the back, and that more weight can be used for Stiff-legged Dead Lifts than for "Good Mornings."

The movement is performed by grasping the bar with the overhand grip at approximately shoulder width. Keeping the elbows and knees completely extended, the back straight, and the head up, the barbell is pulled from the ground until the body is completely erect.

Throwing Exercises

Throwing Motion (Wall Pulley).   A wall pulley is placed above the head or higher and can be used to

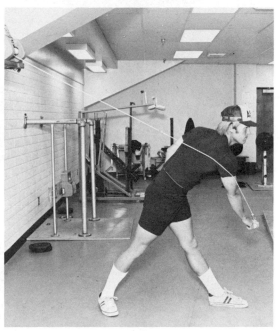

PHOTO 4.30 *Throwing Motion*

increase throwing velocity. It is extremely important that the throwing motion be imitated exactly. Various types of pulleys can be used. Either isotonic or isokinetic ones are effective.

Throwing Pullover. To perform this exercise, a close grip is taken on the bar. The movement is similar to the Bent Arm Pullover in that it is performed in the supine position on a bench, and the bar is brought down to a bent arm position behind and below the head (Picture A, page 78). After the bar is lowered to this position, the power phase of the movement begins. The bar is brought through the movement back to the starting position, with the elbows extended directly above the shoulders. The elbows are held in close to the body throughout the movement. The range of motion closely resembles the throwing motion (Picture B, page 78).

(a)

(b)

PHOTO 4.31   *Throwing Pullover*

Toe Raises

Toe Raises are done to strengthen the calf muscle. The name of this exercise is sometimes misleading because the athlete stands on an elevated support and raises his heels, while the knees are kept straight.

For more complete calf development, the angle of the feet can be adjusted out, straight, or in. This exercise can be done on a calf machine, or upon other devices such as a leg press machine, a Universal Gym bench press, or a military press station.

Standing Tricep Extension

This exercise is done to strength the triceps or elbow extensors. A barbell is used and a close overhand grip is taken. The weight is held directly overhead, with the elbows completely extended. The weight is then lowered behind the head, keeping the elbows close to the head, and then raised again to the starting position (Pictures A and B). This is one of the best methods of isolating the tricep

Tricep Pushdown

The lat machine is used for this exercise, which is done to strengthen the triceps. The athlete stands erect, taking a close grip on the lat bar (Picture A). He or she pulls the bar down to shoulder height (Picture B) and then pushes it straight down as far as possible, using only the arms to move the weight. To keep the tricep isolated, the athlete must not lean or move the shoulders over the bar.

Tricep Supine

This is another method of isolating the tricep. It is done in the supine position upon a bench, using a close grip upon the bar. In the starting position the weight is held directly over the shoulders with the elbows extended. The movement is performed by lowering the weight to the forehead and then back again, not allowing the elbows to slip outward (Pictures A and B, page 81).

Upright Rowing

The shoulders (deltoids and trapezius) and the elbow flexors are strengthened by this exercise. It

(a)

(b)

PHOTO 4.32 *Standing Tricep Extension*

(a)

(b)

PHOTO 4.33   *Tricep Pushdown*

is done by standing erect, with the bar held down in front of the body at arm length (Picture A, page 82). A close grip is used. The movement is performed by flexing the elbows, pulling the bar up to shoulder height and slightly back (Picture B, page 82), then lowering it back to the starting position. The elbows are kept high throughout the movement and the body erect.

SUMMARY

This chapter contains basic information on muscle contractions; types of weight training; the essentials of strength training for athletes; the elements of intensity, frequency, and duration as applied to strength training; and the methods used to devise strength programs. The strength exercises to be used in specific sports programs (Part II) are described and illustrated. The reader is encouraged to refer back to these descriptions in implementing specific conditioning programs for these sports.

REFERENCES

1. Allerheiligen, Bill. "A Basic Program Guide to Beginning, Intermediate, and Advance Strength Cycling." *National Strength and Conditioning Assn. Journal* 4, no. 5 (1982): 33.

2. Anderson, Tim and Kearney, Jay T. "Effects of Three Resistance Training Programs on Muscular Strength and Absolute and Relative Endurance. *Research Quarterly for Exercise and Sport* 53: 1–7 (1982).

3. Battig, W. F. "Facilitation and Interference." In Bilodeau, Edward A. ed., *Acquisition of Skill.* New York: Academic Press, 1969.

4. Berger, Richard. "Effects of Varied Weight Training Programs on Strength." *Research Quarterly* 33 (1962): 168–181.

5. Berger, Richard, and Hardage, Billy. "Effects of Maximum Loads for Each of Ten Repetitions on Strength Improvement." *Research Quarterly* 38 (1967): 715–718.

6. Chui, Edward F. "The Effect of Systematic Weight Training on Athletic Power." *Research Quarterly* 21 (1950): 188–194.

7. Clarke, David H. "Adaptations in Strength and Muscular Endurance Resulting from Exercise." *Exercise & Sports Science Reviews*, vol. 1, pp. 73–102. New York: Academic Press, 1973.

(a)

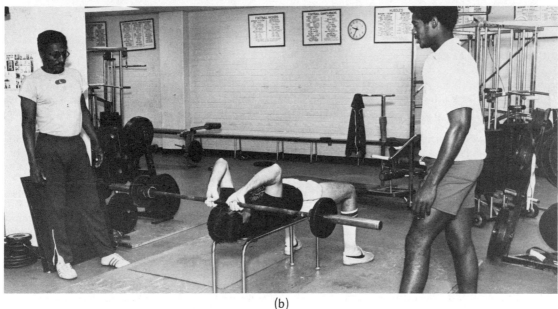

(b)

PHOTO 4.34   *Tricep Supine*

8. Clarke, H. Harrison, ed. "Strength Development and Motor-Sports Improvement." *Physical Fitness Research Digest* 4 (October 1974): 1–17.

9. Counsilman, J. E. "The Importance of Speed in Exercise." *Scholastic Coach* 46 (1976): 94–99.

10. Darden, Ellington. "Misconceptions about Weight Training." *Muscular Development* 9 (1972): 26–27, 48–49.

11. Darden, Ellington. "Weight Training Systems in the U.S.A." *Journal of Physical Education* 70 (1973): 72–76.

12. Dickinson, J. A. *Behavioral Analysis of Sport.* London: Lepus, 1976.

13. Dintiman, George B. *Effects of Various Training Programs on Running Speed. Research Quarterly* 35 (1964): 456.

Dintiman, George B. "Techniques and Methods of Developing Speed in Athletic Performance." *Proceedings: International Symposium on the Art & Science of Coaching*, pp. 97–141. Ontario, Canada: F. I. Productions, 1971.

15. Hoolahan, Paul. "Strength and Conditioning For Basketball: The University of North Carolina Program." *National Strength Coaches Assoc. Journal* 2, no. 4 (Aug.–Sept. 1980): 20–21.

16. Jacobsen, Bert. "Reach Failure to Gain Success." *National Strength and Conditioning Assn. Journal* 3, no. 2 (1981): 24.

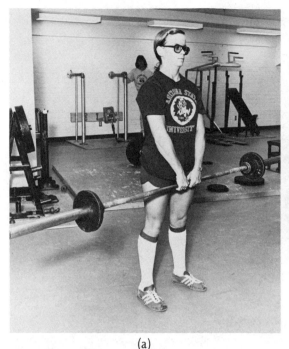

(a)   (b)

PHOTO 4.35 *Upright Rowing*

17. Karpovich, Peter V. "Incidence of Injuries in Weight Lifting." *Journal of Physical Education* 48 (1951): 71–72.
18. Knapp, B. *Skill in Sport.* London: Routledge & Kegan Paul, 1963.
19. Kroll, William A. "An Analysis of the Rate of Strength Development of the Predicted Strength Gain in Collegiate Football Players." *National Strength and Conditioning Assn. Journal* 4, no. 4: 34A (*NSCA Bulletin* 1982).
20. Kroll, William A. "Conditioning for Basketball." *National Strength and Conditioning Assn. Journal* 5, no. 2 (1983): 24.
21. Kroll, William A. "Essentials of Strength Training for Athletes." *National Strength and Conditioning Assn. Journal* 3, no. 4 (Aug.–Sept. 1981): 32–33.
22. Kroll, William A. *Physical Conditioning for Winning Football.* Boston: Allyn and Bacon, 1983.
23. Kroll, William A., and Kroll, Janet. Champaign, IL: Kroll and Kroll *Strength Training Chart.* 1981.
24. Lilian, Gary L. "Optimal Weight Lifting." In *Management Science in Sports.* Vol. 4. Edited by Machol, R. E., Ladnay, Shaul P., and Morrison, Donald G. New York: North Holland Publishing Co., 1976.
25. Moffroid, Mary T., and Whipple, Robert H. *Specificity of Speed Exercises.* U.S. Public Health Service, Grant FR 00291, 1970.
26. Murray, James, and Karpovich, Peter V. *Weight Training in Athletics.* Englewood Cliffs, N.J.: Prentice-Hall, 1956.
27. O'Shea, Patrick J. *Scientific Principles and Methods of Strength Fitness,* 2d ed. Reading, Mass.: Addison-Wesley, 1976.
28. Pedemonte, Jimmy. "Training of General, Specific and Special Strength: A Key to Improved Performances in Sport." *National Strength and Conditioning Assn. Journal* 3, no. 6 (1981): 54.
29. Rasch, Philip J. *Weight Training,* 4th ed. Dubuque, Iowa: William C. Brown Co., 1982.
30. Starck, Al. "Abuse of the Overload Principle: A Physiological Basis for Cycling." *National Strength and Conditioning Assn. Journal* 4, no. 1 (1982): 36.
31. Vermeil, Al, and Chu, Don. "Periodization of Strength Training for Professional Football." *National Strength and Conditioning Assn. Journal* 4, no. 3 (1982): 54.
32. Westcott, Wayne L. "Effects of Varied Frequencies of Weight Training on the Development of Strength." Master's thesis, Pennsylvania State University, 1974.
33. Westcott, Wayne L. *Strength Fitness: Physiological Principles and Training Techniques.* Boston: Allyn and Bacon, 1982.
34. Wickstrom, Ralph L. "Weight Training and Flexibility." *JOHPER,* Feb. 1963, p. 61.
35. Wilmore, Jack H. *Athletic Training and Physical Fitness,* 2d ed. Boston: Allyn and Bacon, 1983.
36. Zorbas, William S., and Karpovich, Peter V. "The Effect of Weight Lifting upon the Speed of Muscular Contractions." *Research Quarterly* 22 (1951): 145–148.

5

Flexibility, Warm-Up, and Stretching

In the first edition of this book the authors stressed the importance and necessity of stretching exercises for athletes. It was recommended that stretching be conducted both pre– and post–exercise, either in practice or in competition. Unfortunately, very little space was allotted to the concepts of flexibility, stretching, and warming-up. In the intervening years stretching exercises have become very much "in vogue" for athletes at all levels of competition. Stretching has become a very common pre-event ritual for the 10K weekend runner as well as the professional athlete in team sports. Warming-up and stretching are not entirely new practices for athletes, but a serious examination of those techniques is fairly recent.

While it is gratifying to the authors to see increased attention to stretching as a part of preparation for sport, it is also evident that confusion has developed concerning the relationships between warming-up, stretching exercises, and flexibility. A number of stretching and flexibility systems appear to be vying for prominence in sport. As so often occurs in scientific study, it may be that several systems are effective in developing flexibility. It is clear to the authors that there is a need to distinguish between the objectives of warming-up exercises versus stretching exercises, even when they are done together as was suggested in the earlier edition of this book. The authors have added this chapter in order to address the very questions and problems indicated above. Also included is a greatly expanded list of stretching exercises and some suggested stretching programs.

FLEXIBILITY

Flexibility is the range of motion in a joint or series of joints. Most interest in flexibility in the past has involved physical therapy or other medically related applications designed to rehabilitate patients. Flexibility has also been recognized recently as one of the components of physical fitness. Two kinds of flexibility have been distinguished, static flexibility and dynamic flexibility. Static flexibility is determined by measuring the range of motion (ROM) about a joint or series of joints. The body is not in motion, nor is there any effort to move quickly as the ROM of a joint is measured "statically." An example would be to reach slowly toward the toes with the knees straight, in a sitting position (the sit and reach). Dynamic flexibility, on the other hand, implies moving flexibility and may also involve high speed action. The simultaneous leap and kick of the dancer is an example of dynamic flexibility. It should be evident that most athletic events involve dynamic ROM.

Flexibility is usually measured in the static mode and a variety of instruments have been used to measure it. The simplest instrument for measuring flexibility has been the goniometer, which measures the angle of the ROM. The elgon, or electrogoniometer, is a more sophisticated instrument which can also measure dynamic flexibility angles. The Leighton flexometer can be strapped onto a limb and can measure the ROM in slow or rapid movement.[13] Sit-and-reach type tests, or floor-touch tests, have also been used as screening tests for flexibility and require no sophisticated equipment.

The Nature of Flexibility

A number of anatomic factors determine flexibility. The most important factor, for stretching programs, is the muscles. Flexibility at a joint will be reduced if the muscles operating at the joint are tight or shortened. This can occur from lack of use or overuse and also from emotional anxiety, which can lead to muscular tension. The myotatic stretch reflex of the muscle also operates when the muscle is rapidly stretched, as in the knee jerk. The rapidly stretching muscle sends messages to the nervous system, which quickly signals the muscle to contract. In the tight or shortened muscle the stretch reflex will operate early as the muscle is stretched and thus inhibit stretch. The stretch reflex is responsible for protecting the muscle from a rapid stretch and possible tear or injury. When the stretch reflex is engaged early in the stretch, the stretched muscle contracts, and full stretch and relaxation are impossible. The muscle is fighting against itself in such situations.

The connective tissue in and around the joint is also responsible for determining flexibility. In addition to the muscle, ligaments, the joint capsule itself and tendons are also influential in determining flexibility.[12] The more elastic the joint connective tissue is, the greater is the ROM. It is important to note, however, that most efforts to increase flexibility through stretching are directed to the muscle. Ligaments and tendons do not have the elasticity of muscle tissue; hence it is undesirable to produce too much slack in them. If they become overstretched or injured, their ability to maintain the integrity of the joint is greatly reduced. Although there are no clear standards for optimal flexibility at this time, no particular advantage comes from possessing "excessive" flexibility. Excessive flexibility in the joint might even be associated with a higher potential for joint injury.

One of the proposed causes of muscle injuries is a lack of flexibility. The tight or shortened muscle that has not relaxed, or that is in a state of myotatic stretch reflex, may be more susceptible to injury or tear. It is frequently suggested that the unyielding antagonist, such as a thin hamstring, is overpowered and injured by the more powerful agonist, in this case the quadriceps group. In a cold or unrelaxed state the tight muscle would be more prone to injury. Unfortunately, there is not a great deal of clinical or experimental data to confirm the suggestion. It would certainly appear prudent at this time to maintain flexibility and avoid practices that tighten or shorten the muscle.

Certain factors associated with flexibility do give us additional information about its nature. For some time it has been known that flexibility tends to decrease with age, even in children. It has also been noted that females tend to be more flexible than males.[14] The precise reasons for sex differences are unknown, but they could be attributed to different activity patterns. Body build, on the other hand, does not appear to contribute to differences in flexibility.

One of the most firmly established characteristics of flexibility is its specificity.[5] This means that in any individual, good shoulder flexibility may not be accompanied by good knee flexibility. The same joint on one side of the body may be more or less flexible than its counterpart on the other side of the body. This also implies that there is no general characteristic of flexibility. Level of activity has been associated with flexibility, and it may also contribute to some of the specific patterns of flexibility for individuals or groups. As a result, stretching will aid only the joints being stretched.

Efforts to increase flexibility through stretching programs have been successful. Greater ROM can result through systematic stretching programs.[5] Athletes generally are more flexible than nonathletic groups, but there are differences among sports groups. Baseball players and swimmers have been found to be very flexible, weight lifters are more flexible than normal, while wrestlers tend to be less flexible among athletic groups. Within sports groups specific patterns of flexibility are related to frequent or unique joint movements in those sports.

The effects of increased flexibility on sports performance may range from obvious to subtle. There is face validity to the need for excellent flexibility in dance, gymnastics, diving, and swimming. Those sports have an aesthetic component, and increased flexibility obviously enhances performance since it is part of the scoring system. The contributions of flexibility to the performance in many team sports is less obvious. Athletes in baseball, basketball, football, and other team sports frequently exhibit excellent flexibility. Their performances may be aesthetically pleasing, especially in slow-motion instant replay, but they are judged solely on effect—did the player catch the ball or make the basket? A few efforts have been made to relate flexibility to physical performance, and they have generally been successful as long as the flexibility is specific to the sports event.[6]

Temperature, both environmental and internal, appears to have an effect on flexibility. Flexibility seems to be enhanced in a warm environment; most athletes have experienced that effect. In addition, some warm-up or prior stretch results in better flexibility when it is subsequently measured. The effects of warming-up and its relationship to stretching and flexibility are also important to understand.

WARM-UP

Stretching exercises do not necessarily warm up the athlete. Their purpose is to relax and lengthen the muscle through stretching and, eventually, to increase flexibility. Warming-up, on the other hand, serves to increase blood flow, elevate the temperature of the muscle, and lubricate the joints via joint fluids. In the whole body sense, warm-up also serves to elevate metabolism by increasing heart rate, respiratory rate, and oxygen uptake.[3] As indicated above, warming-up also serves to increase flexibility, since flexibility is enhanced in heated muscles. Some observers have even suggested that a warm-up period should be done *prior to* stretching.[16]

Warming-up exercises can consist of rhythmic calisthenics and jogging, if the main purpose is to elevate metabolism and warm the muscles. Warm-up exercises can precede stretching or be combined with stretching. Warming-up exercises should gradually increase in vigor just as repeated stretching seeks to lengthen the muscle more with each effort. The value of warming-up is not without some controversy, and it is appropriate here to review the information available about warm-up.

The effects of warm-up listed above are not controversial. The effects on muscles, joints, and metabolism are rather clear. The established benefits of reduced injury or greater safety for exercising adults are not well documented. The objectives of warming the muscles, based on physiological effects, are primarily related to reduced injury potential, increased flexibility, and better performance. Adults are also cautioned to

undergo whole body warm-up to elevate metabolism and to prepare their cardiorespiratory system for more intense activity. There are also questions to be raised about the nature of the warm-up and the subsequent performance, as well as injury and safety.

Many different warming-up techniques have been employed in studies of warm-up.[15] Nonspecific (unrelated) and even passive techniques have not proved effective in improving performance. They would include hot showers, message, local heating, and mild calisthenics. Specific (related) and more vigorous types of warm-ups have generally had a positive effect on performance. They usually involve a vigorous period of actual practice of the sport skill. Much of the value of actual practice of a motor skill prior to competition involves a renewal of the psychomotor skill. This is evident in such things as the baseball pitcher's warm-up, batting practice, basketball pre-game shooting, and other related practice. For those events that require more strength, power, aerobic, or anaerobic effort than skill, the vigor of the warm-up appears to be important. In such cases the pre-event warm-up should be vigorous enough to produce the physiological effects mentioned above. This means elevated muscle and/or body temperature. Perhaps no area of exercise science has been so thoroughly studied yet remains so controversial as the area of warm-up. Since the preponderance of evidence, both research and clinical, supports warm-up, the authors recommend that it follow the guidelines above.

One last point to be discussed about warm-up involves the time sequence. Depending upon the environment, the effects of warming-up can be expected to last approximately one-half hour and should be planned accordingly. A lengthy period of inactivity (sitting on the bench, or half-time rest) will result in a cooling-off. Additional warm-up and stretching are required in such instances. In very cold weather the warm-up effect may not last thirty minutes; in hot weather it may last much longer.

STRETCHING

Stretching has both a short-term and a long-term effect. The short-term effects include increased ROM, lengthening and relaxing the muscle, and reducing the soreness and/or injury potential. These are the reasons for stretching pre- and post-exercise. These objectives are related to flexibility, but increased flexibility does not permanently occur after a few stretching sessions. The long-term effect of repeated stretching sessions, done in relation to exercise or at other times, is an increase in flexibility. The evidence is discussed in greater detail above, but it is important to note the distinction between the long-term and short-term effects of stretching. Both of those effects have potential for improved performance.

Ballistic Stretching

Many different stretching techniques have been employed over the years. Most of them have proved effective in increasing flexibility. They can generally be assigned to two categories of stretch: ballistic or static. Static stretches involve slow movement and a held stretch in the extended position. Ballistic stretching includes those rapid stretching movements that are characterized as "bouncing" or "bobbing." Rapid bends to a toe touch are an example of ballistic stretching. Some vigorous warm-up calisthenics involve ballistic stretch. Preparation for vigorous activity, as has been established previously, requires a vigorous warm-up, often of the actual event. Flexibility programs that have used ballistic stretching have proved successful in increasing flexibility.[6] Despite that success, most sports scientists recommend static stretching programs because they are less likely to produce the myotatic stretch reflex.

Static Stretching

The term *static stretching* is usually associated with the work of deVries.[7, 8] The technique involves a slow stretch and "hold" of the stretched position from several seconds to a minute. The major advantage of the static stretch technique is that it will not elicit the myotatic stretch reflex if done properly. A major reason for increasing the length of muscles—and hence flexibility—is to avoid the stretch reflex. The tight or shortened muscle will respond with contraction to rapid stretch. This suggests that ballistic stretching, although generally effective, is stretching a muscle in partial contraction. This is ineffective in producing a full ROM and totally ineffective in relaxing the muscle. The very technique employed (ballistic) to reduce injury could also lead to injury—and it has.

Most static stretching adherents emphasize the importance of *relaxing* the stretched muscle.[1, 4, 17] Relaxation enables the stretched muscle to cease stretch reflex impulses coming from the muscle spindles. Anderson recommends a technique that involves two parts.[1] First the muscle is stretched in the *easy* stage for 20 to 30 seconds. By this time the muscle should have relaxed and the stretch reflex halted. The easy stage is followed by a *developmental* stage, which involves an added stretch-and-hold for 30 seconds. At no time does the technique involve a drastic or painful stretch, and the entire period of stretch involves 50 to 60 seconds. Anderson's technique is highly applicable to sport, and he illustrates specialized stretching programs for specific sports.[1]

ACS. While static stretching adherents agree on the use of the slow, relaxed stretch, they differ slightly on the application of the stretch. Shelton, a pioneer in developing flexibility programs for therapeutic as well as athletic purposes, recommends an Active Controlled Stretch (ACS).[17] The starting position is important in ACS as the muscle to be stretched should be in a gravity-assisted position. When the biceps is contracted (flexion at the elbow) in the standing position, it is in an anti-gravity position and the triceps can be stretched and relaxed in a gravity-assisted position. In that same position it is difficult to stretch the biceps or get it to relax, since it is constantly counteracting gravity (anti-gravity).

Shelton maintains that the two-joint muscles are more susceptible to shortening and tightening.[17] They include, among anothers, the hamstrings and the gastrocnemius (calf). Shelton also suggests the addition of manual assistance if the contracting muscle is not strong enough to adequately stretch the tight muscle. A great deal of caution must be advised, since manual assistance is usually a therapeutic technique and too vigorous a push can trigger the stretch reflex or injure the muscle. The authors do not recommend the use of manual assistance when it is employed by young athletes with limited knowledge of anatomy. The person using manual assistance to a stretch must be quick to reverse the movement when the stretched muscle produces a myotatic stretch reflex.

PNF. Proprioceptive Neuromuscular Facilitation (PNF) is primarily a therapeutic technique that has found its way into sport stretching programs.[9, 11] The technique is similar to ACS with some slight variation. The muscle to be stretched is first placed on a slight stretch and then contracted isometrically. After a few seconds the muscle is relaxed and then stretched by action of the opposite muscle, as in ACS. A partner is used in PNF to serve as resistance for the isometric contraction and to apply manual assistance during the lengthening stretch. A six-count sequence is used for both the contraction and the stretch, and each stretch is done twice. Again the authors recommend caution in using partner-assisted stretching. Static stretching and ACS can be accomplished without the use of a partner.

STRETCHING PRINCIPLES

Other stretching techniques, including Yoga and Kung Fu, have been used in sports flexibility programs. The name of the stretching technique is less important than the application of sound stretching principles.

1. The purpose of stretching is to lengthen and relax the muscle and ultimately increase flexibility. Like strength, there will always be individual differences in flexibility, thus flexibility training should not be a contest.[1] Stretching programs should be individualized as much as possible.
2. Slow, static stretching is recommended. When the stretch is held for 30 to 60 seconds, it gives time for the muscle to relax and the stretch reflex to dissipate, both pre- or post-activity.
3. Warming-up requires vigorous related activity to be effective. The purpose of warm-up is to elevate muscle and body temperature as well as metabolism. Vigorous ballistic activity may be part of the warm-up.
4. Since flexibility is specific, the application of stretching exercises should include specific muscle groups used in your sport or event. Some general flexibility exercises should be done for each of the major areas of the body, starting from the head and working down: neck, upper body, trunk, back, and legs.

WARM-UP AND STRETCHING EXERCISES

Warm-Up Exercises

Warm-up exercises, as previously indicated, are most effective if they are vigorous and actually

related to the activity to follow. Several warm-up exercises are listed below, and they are designed to cover whole body warm-up. Specific, task-related warm-ups are suggested, just as the athlete should select stretching exercises that are aimed at specific joints and muscles involved in subsequent practice or competition.

Deep Breathing

From a standing position, inhale fully as the arms are raised in front to the overhead position. Exhale fully as the arms are lowered to the sides. Repeat 10 times.

Arm Circles

Extend arms to the side, shoulder height. Rotate

PHOTO 5.1 *Deep Breathing*

PHOTO 5.2 *Arm Circles*

arms in tight (6") circles, reversing direction after 10 counts. Repeat twice.

Chest Stretcher

Extend arms forward, shoulder height. Pull arms back vigorously with bobbing motion and four counts. Extend arms to the front and repeat 5 to 10 times.

Burpee

Bend over and place hands on floor directly in front of feet. With weight on hands, thrust legs straight out to the back. From this arm support position, thrust feet back to original position and stand erect. Repeat 5 to 10 times.

Jumping Jacks

From standing position, jump up and bring arms over head to the sides as feet spread to the side. Return to starting position on the second count. This exercise should be done rapidly to a 1-2-3-4 count. Repeat 5 to 10 counts of 1-2-3-4.

PHOTO 5.3 *Chest Stretcher*

PHOTO 5.4　*Burpee*

Running-in-Place

Start with a slow jog-in-place, gradually increasing the speed and height of knee action. Running-in-place can continue for 1 to 3 minutes.

Stretching—Whole Body

The stretching exercises below have been organized into stretches for different areas of the body. The coach or athlete should select stretching exercises for all the major areas of the body, while also selecting specific stretches that work the muscles and joints involved in the specific sport.

Relaxation Stretch

Lying on the back, gradually relax all areas of the body. Begin by shaking loosely the hands, ankles, arms, legs until the entire body is loosened and relaxed. All of the body parts should become limp and relaxed with a feeling of great heaviness. This is an excellent technique for getting complete relaxation prior to competition as well as for relaxing the muscles and making them less resistant to stretching.

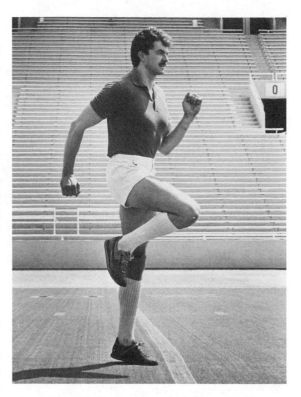

PHOTO 5.5   *Running in Place*

PHOTO 5.6   *Relaxation Stretch*

STRETCHING—
NECK AND UPPER BODY

Neck Rotation

From a standing position, rotate the head very slowly in one direction for 4 counts. Reverse direction for 4 counts. Repeat 2 to 3 times in each direction.

Tricep and Shoulder Stretch

This stretch is done in the standing position. First, the arms are extended straight overhead so that the inside of the elbow is next to the head. (See Photo 5.8, Picture A.) Then reach across and grasp the elbow of the arm and shoulder to be stretched. The elbow is flexed and then slowly pulled behind the head until the shoulder and tricep stretch is felt. (See Photo 5.8, Picture B.)

Shoulder and Side Stretch

This stretch is done from the same position as the "tricep and shoulder stretch." The upper arm is held against the head. (See Photo 5.9.) The stretch is then done by bending sideways from the hip, stretching the muscles of the side and rib cage.

PHOTO 5.7 *Neck Rotation*

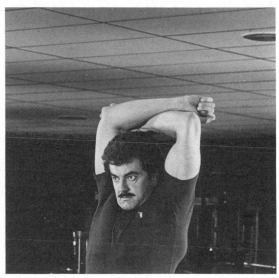

(a)   (b)

PHOTO 5.8 *Tricep and Shoulder Stretch*

PHOTO 5.9   *Shoulder and Side Stretch*

Shoulder and Chest Stretch

This exercise is done in the standing position by first interlocking the fingers behind the back. (See Photo 5.10, Picture A.) Then bend forward, keeping the elbows straight and lifting the arms as high as possible. (See Photo 5.10, Picture B.) This can

(a)

(b)

(c)

PHOTO 5.10   *Shoulder and Chest Stretch*

be done with the palms either up or down. (See Photo 5.10, Picture C.)

extended behind him while the assistant holds the wrists and lifts them gently until the stretch is felt in the shoulders and/or chest.

Assisted Chest and Shoulder Stretch

This stretch can also be performed from the sitting position with an assistant. The athlete's arms are

Overhead Shoulder Stretch

From standing position, extend the arms in front

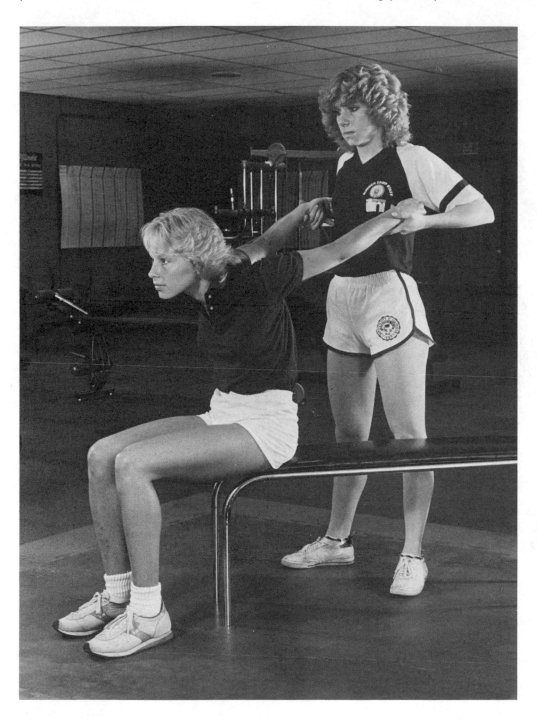

PHOTO 5.11   *Assisted Chest and Shoulder Stretch*

(a)   (b)

PHOTO 5.12 *Overhead Shoulder Stretch*

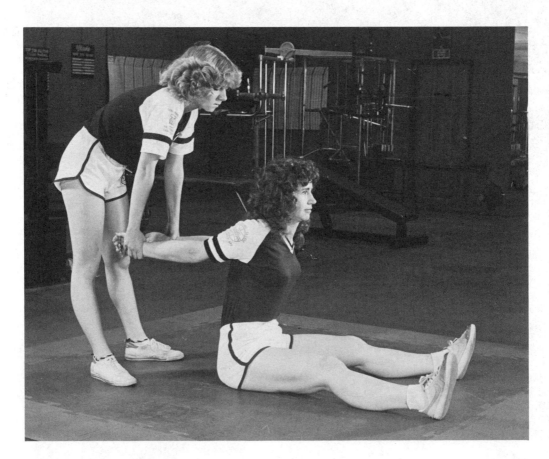

PHOTO 5.13 *Assisted PNF Shoulder and Chest Stretch*

of the body, interlocking the fingers (see Photo 5.12, Picture A) and turning the palms outward (see Photo 5.12, Picture B). Raise the arms overhead until the stretch is felt.

Assisted PNF Shoulder and Chest Stretch

The athlete begins in the sitting position with the assistant standing behind him. The arms are extended behind him with the elbows kept straight and the thumbs pointed upward. The assistant grasps the athlete's wrists and applies "easy" pressure, pulling the arms together. The athlete attempts to move the arms in the opposite direction on the "flex" command. On "stretch" the assistant applies the inward pressure, repeating the stretch until the developmental stretch is felt.

STRETCHING—TRUNK AND GROIN

Side Bends

From a standing position, bend to the side with a *slow*, stretching motion as the arm reaches down the side of the leg. Hold position and relax. Alternate stretching one side and then the other. Repeat five times each side.

Trunk Rotation

Standing with hands on hips, rotate slowly from the waist, with legs straight. Rotate four counts in one direction and then reverse for four counts

PHOTO 5.14 *Side Bends*

PHOTO 5.15 *Trunk Rotation*

or rotations. Repeat two to three full four counts on each side.

Standing Groin Stretch

The exercise is begun by first stepping to the side in one direction to achieve a wide stance. The groin is then stretched in the traditional way by bending the right leg at the knee while shifting the body weight over the right leg, keeping the left knee extended, thus stretching the inside part of the left leg (see Photo 5.16, Picture B).

From this "wide stance" position, the back toe is then pointed toward the opposite foot. The knee is then flexed in the same manner as before, stretching the front part of the upper thigh and hip as well as the calf and hamstring.

This stretch can be extended into the "splits" stretch. From the wide stance position described

(a)

(b)

PHOTO 5.16   *Standing Groin Stretch*

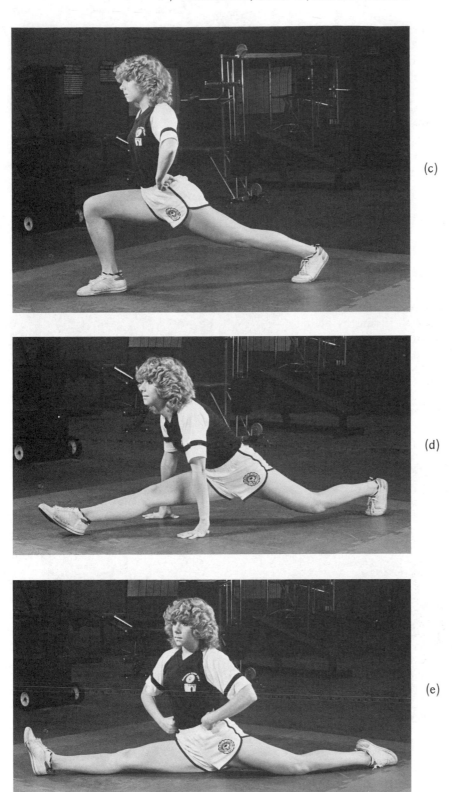

(c)

(d)

(e)

PHOTO 5.16 *Standing Groin Stretch (Continued)*

above, the stance is widened. As the hips are lowered, the hands are placed on the floor for balance. The toe of the front foot is pointed upward with the heel on the floor (see Photo 5.16, Picture D). At first the full split position is difficult to achieve. Later, more flexibility can be attained, staying within the developmental stretch (see Photo 5.16, Picture E).

The Yogi

This exercise is particularly good in preventing groin pulls and strains. It is done in the sitting position by bringing the legs to a crossed position (Indian style), then placing the bottoms of the feet together. In this position the feet are kept close to the buttocks, and the stretch is done by pushing the knees down toward the floor. An advanced method is to have an assistant help develop flexibility in this area by placing a greater stretch on the area by pushing on the knees. This method is used by many high school and collegiate wrestlers

PHOTO 5.17   *The Yogi*

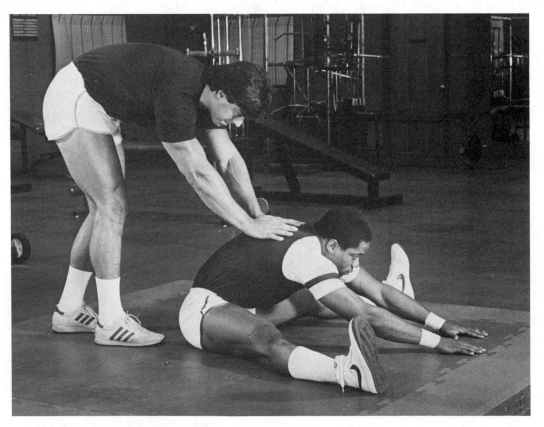

PHOTO 5.18   *Assisted PNF Lower Back and Groin Stretch*

and must be developed by slowly increasing the pressure over a number of training sessions.

Assisted PNF Lower Back and Groin Stretch

From the sitting position, with the legs as wide as possible, the athlete bends forward at the waist until an "easy" stretch is felt in the lower back and/or groin. The assistant then stands behind the athlete and places the hands just below the shoulder blades. On the "flex" command the athlete flexes the lower back by attempting to return the torso to the upright sitting position while the assistant provides resistance. The stretch is done by bending forward at the waist, the assistant adding the additional movement until the developmental stretch is achieved.

Assisted PNF Sitting Groin Stretch

The athlete takes the sitting position with the legs spread as wide as possible. A slight bend at the knee is permissible. The assistant places the hands inside the athlete's knees to provide resistance.

The athlete attempts to push the legs together on the "flex" command. On the "stretch" command the assistant stretches the groin by placing pressure in the opposite direction.

Assisted PNF Lying Groin Stretch

The athlete performs this stretch by lying on the back with the legs extended straight upward and held apart. The assistant stands with the shins against the back of the athlete's thighs and places the hands on the inside of the athlete's knees. On "ready," the athlete attempts to spread the legs as far as possible. On the "flex" command the athlete attempts to bring the legs together. The athlete is permitted only slight movement before the isometric contraction. The stretch is done by the athlete again, attempting to spread the legs as wide as possible while the assistant continues the movement until the developmental stretch is achieved.

Assisted PNF Hip Flexor Stretch

The athlete lies face down and bends the right leg at the knee so that the lower leg is perpendicular

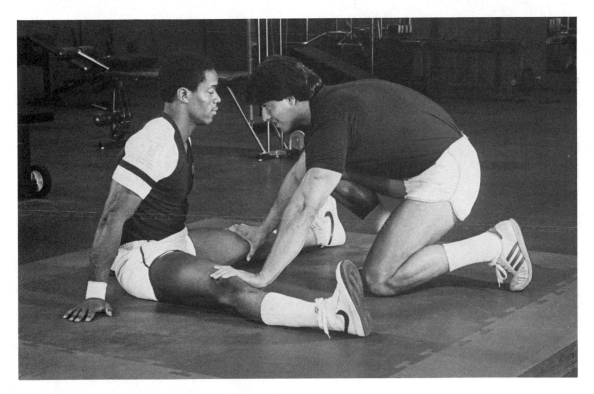

PHOTO 5.19   *Assisted PNF Sitting Groin Stretch*

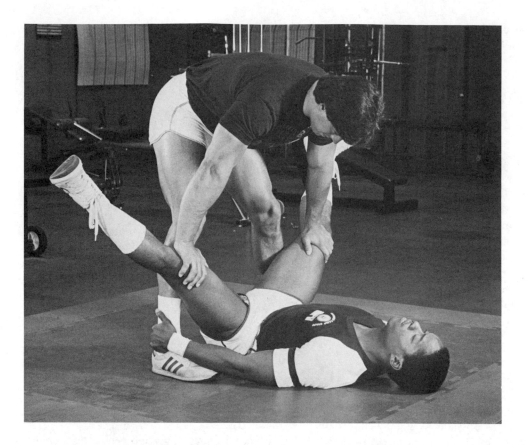

PHOTO 5.20   *Assisted PNF Lying Groin Stretch*

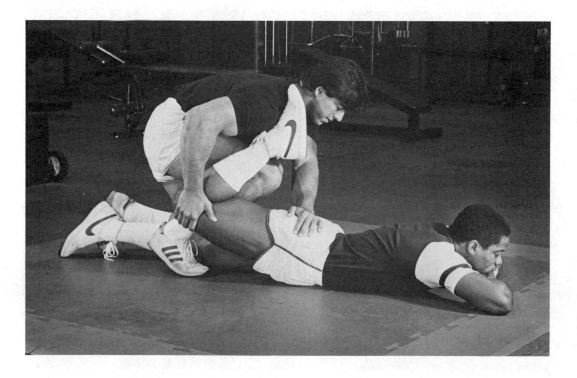

PHOTO 5.21   *Assisted PNF Hip Flexor Stretch*

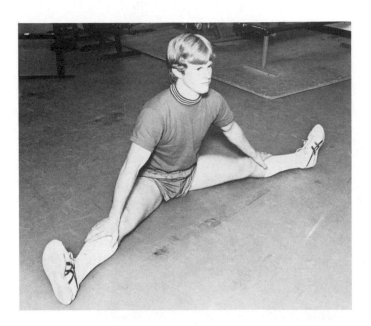

PHOTO 5.22   *Wide Straddle Seat*

to the ground. The assistant kneels behind the athlete and places the athlete's ankle on the right shoulder and the right hand under the athlete's right knee. The assistant puts the left hand on the athlete's right buttock and holds it down while lifting the right knee so that the hip flexor receives an "easy" stretch. When the "flex" command is given, the athlete attempts to drive the right knee down to the ground. The assistant resists. On the "stretch" command the assistant lifts the knee again, holding the buttock down until the hip flexor receives a developmental stretch. The stretch is performed twice for each hip.

Wide Straddle Seat

From the seated position, with the head and back erect, the legs are spread as far as possible for the stretch. Keeping the torso erect, the athlete leans forward, stretching the groin and hamstrings. The stretch is then held for 10 or more seconds, relaxed, and repeated.

STRETCHING—BACK AND LEGS

Head-to-Knee Stretch

This stretch is done from the sitting position. It stretches the lower back and hamstrings. The bottom of one foot is placed against the upper inside thigh of the opposite leg (see Photo 5.23, Picture A). The foot of the extended leg is kept with the toe pointing straight up. The athlete sits up perfectly straight and then begins the stretch by bending forward at the waist. The athlete stretches by leaning forward at the waist only, not by lowering the head and reaching for the toe (see Photo 5.23, Picture B). This exercise can also be done with the flexed leg in the hurdler's position (See Photo 5.23, Picture C). The stretch from this position is not as direct and stretches the hamstring and lower back in a slightly different way.

Bending Forward Stretch

This exercise, which stretches the lower back and hamstrings, is done in the standing position. Variations are done with the legs together or apart. The head is lowered to the knees until tightness is felt. This position is held for 30 to 60 seconds. Return to the standing position and relax for several seconds; then repeat the exercise. The hands and arms may be used to help pull the head toward the knees. This should be done easily at first with light to moderately firm pressure.[7]

Foot-to-Hand Stretch

This exercise stretches the muscles of the hips and lower back. It is done in the supine position with

(a)

(b)

(c)

PHOTO 5.23   *Head-to-Knee Stretch*

PHOTO 5.24   *Bending Forward Stretch*

the arms extended perpendicular to the sides of the body. In the starting position the legs are together. Keeping the knees straight, one leg is moved diagonally across, flexing and rotating the hip until the foot touches the opposite hand. After the stretch the leg is returned to the starting position. After several seconds of rest the stretch is repeated with the other leg. As a variation, stretching slightly different muscles can be done by using both legs instead of only one. As in all stretches, if the extreme or complete position cannot be attained immediately, it should be of no concern.[7]

Lying Hamstring Stretch

Lying on back, raise one leg as high as possible over head with knee straight. Hold stretch. Repeat

exercise with opposite leg and complete 5 reps with each leg.

Back Stretcher

Take position on hands and knees with back straight. Slide backwards until sitting on heels with palms still on floor, arms straight, head down. Return to starting position while arching back slightly. Repeat 5 times.

Low-Back Stretch

Lying on back, grab below one knee with both hands. Bring knee to chest, holding 30 to 60 seconds. Repeat with other leg. Then bring both

PHOTO 5.25   *Foot-to-Hand Stretch*

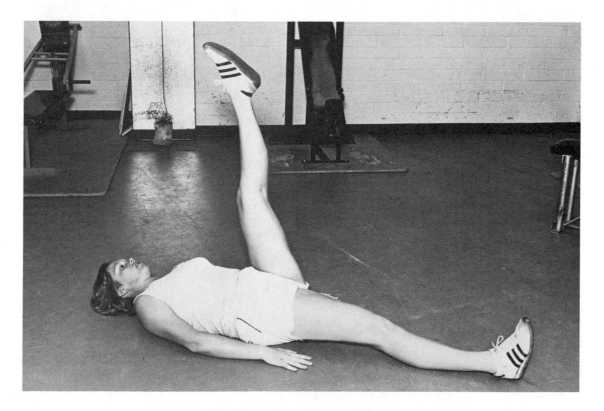

PHOTO 5.26   *Lying Hamstring Stretch*

PHOTO 5.27   *Back Stretcher*

PHOTO 5.28   *Low-Back Stretch*

legs up to chest and hold again 30 to 60 seconds. Repeat 5 to 10 times.

Hanging Stretch

Many athletes, especially football linemen, can benefit from hanging from a bar. The time of the hang can be increased gradually from a few seconds up to one minute. This exercise helps stretch the vertebral joints. It relieves pressure on the discs

between the vertebrae, and stretches the muscles of the back, the shoulders, the rib cage, and the sides.

Head-to-Knee and Chest-to-Floor
(from the wide straddle seat position)

This exercise stretches the hamstrings and lower back. It is done with the seated straddle position as the starting point. Other variations are done

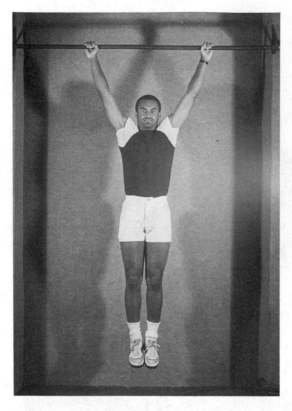

PHOTO 5.29 *Hanging Stretch*

with the legs together, or from the "hurdles position."

Assisted PNF Hamstring Stretch

The athlete being stretched lies on the back and raises the right leg straight upward, perpendicular to the ground. The assistant kneels and puts the hands on the athlete's knee, to be sure that it is kept straight during the stretch. The chest and shoulder are placed against the athlete's ankles and calf (see Photo 5.31).

On the "ready" command the athlete locks the knee and flexes the hip as far as possible. On the "flex" command the athlete flexes the hamstring while the assistant resists, allowing only slight movement. On "stretch," the athlete flexes the hip while the assistant applies gradual pressure until the developmental stretch is achieved. The stretch is done twice on each hamstring.

Quadricep Stretch

This stretch is done from the hurdler's position

(a) *Head-to-Knee*

(b) *Chest-to-Floor*

PHOTO 5.30

PHOTO 5.31   *Assisted PNF Hamstring Stretch*

(a)

(b)

PHOTO 5.32   *Quadricep Stretch*

PHOTO 5.33   *Prone Quadricep Stretch*

with one leg bent and the other extended. See Photo 5.32 where the right leg is being stretched.

It can also be performed with the opposite knee flexed by placing the bottom of the foot of the leg not being stretched on the inside of the upper thigh (see Photo 5.32, Picture B). The ankle of the leg being stretched should be extended with the front of the ankle touching the floor. The foot should not be allowed to point out to the side with the inside of the foot and/or ankle against the floor. This tends to weaken the knee, placing an undesirable stress on the inside of the knee.[1]

Prone Quadricep Stretch

Lying prone, the athlete bends the knee and grasps behind the ankle with the arm on the same side. Stretch slowly and hold for 30 to 60 seconds. Repeat with opposite leg after returning to original position. Repeat 3 to 5 times.

STRETCHING—LOWER LEGS

Calf Stretch

This exercise is done by leaning against a wall, pole, or some other stationary object. From the standing position, approximately 3½ to 4½ feet from the wall, the athlete faces the wall and then leans against the wall, keeping the heels flat on the ground. The feet should be pointed straight ahead (see Photo 5.34). One knee is then raised as close as possible toward the chest, placing a greater stretch on the calf muscles of the opposite leg. This is done with both legs and then repeated. Taller persons will need to stand farther from the wall. If an object to lean against is not available, this stretch can be done by placing one foot ahead of the other and then leaning forward, keeping the feet pointed straight ahead with the heel down (see Photo 5.34).

Ankle Stretch

The ankle can be stretched in the sitting position by flexing the knee, grasping the foot, and then stretching the foot manually through each of its movements. They include rotation in both directions, flexion, extension, inversion, and eversion.

Heel Cord Stretch

In sitting position with legs straight, curl toes toward body. Hold stretch for 30 to 60 seconds, maintaining straight legs. Repeat 3 to 5 times.

Assisted PNF Ankle Stretcher

The ankle is stretched in four directions: flexion, extension, inversion, and eversion. This stretch is done with the athlete lying on the back while the assistant stands at the feet. The foot is grasped by the assistant and placed in the stretched posi-

PHOTO 5.34 *Calf Stretch*

PHOTO 5.35 *Ankle Stretch*

PHOTO 5.36 *Heel Cord Stretch*

tion. On the "flex" command the athlete attempts to straighten the ankle and the assistant offers resistance. When the "stretch" command is given, the assistant moves the ankle to the point where the developmental stretch is received. The stretch is done on each ankle twice for each of the four directions. This is the most time-consuming of the stretches and may be abbreviated by stretching in two of the directions per day on alternate days.

STRETCHING PROGRAMS

Several sample stretching programs are listed below. They are intended to be illustrative of whole body stretching and are related to the kind of conditioning anticipated or completed (see Figures 5.1 to 5.5 on page 113). Specialized programs for specific sports or specific events should be developed by the coach or the athlete. Examples of football and basketball stretching programs are included.

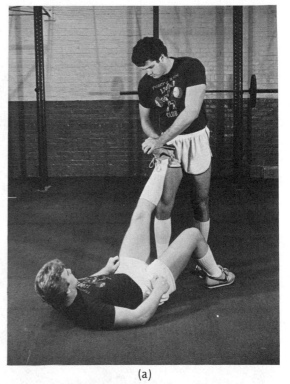

(a)

PHOTO 5.37 *Assisted PNF Ankle Stretch*

SUMMARY

Stretching and flexibility exercises have become important aspects of preparing the athlete for practice and competition. Warming-up, which can

(b)   (c)

(d)   (e)

PHOTO 3.37

precede stretching, is designed to elevate muscle temperature and body metabolism. Stretching exercises have the short-term effect of relaxing and lengthening the muscle. Habitual stretching leads to increased flexibility, and the preferred technique is the slow or static stretching routine. Stretching exercises should not only focus on the major areas of the body but also involve sport-specific stretching to match the anticipated movements of the event.

REFERENCES

1. Anderson, Robert A. *Stretching*. Palmer Lake, CO: Stretching, 1980.
2. Beaulieu, John E. *Stretching for All Sports*. N. Palm Beach, FL: Athletic Institute, 1981.
3. Benjamin, Ben E. "Creating Your Own Warm-up." *Dance Magazine* 54 (November 1980): 86–88.
4. Benjamin, Ben E. "The Do's and Don'ts of Stretching." *Dance Magazine* 54 (December 1980): 88–89.
5. Clarke, H. Harrison, ed. "Joint and Body Range of

Movement." _Physical Fitness Research Digest_ 5 (October, 1975): 1–22.

6. Corbin, Charles B., and Noble, Larry. "Flexibility: A Major Component of Physical Fitness." _JOPER_ 51 (June 1980): 23–24, 57–60.

7. deVries, Herbert A. "Flexibility, an Overlooked but Vital Factor in Sports Conditioning." _Proceedings: International Symposium on the Art and Science of Coaching_, pp. 209–221. Ontario, Canada: F. I. Productions, 1971.

8. deVries, Herbert A. _The Physiology of Exercise for Physical Education and Athletics._ 3d ed. Dubuque, IA: William C. Brown Co., 1980.

9. Houglum, Peggy. "Techniques of P.N.F. in Athletic Training." _Athletic Training_ 10 (March 1975): 44–45.

10. Jensen, Clayne. "Pertinent Facts About Warm-up." _The Athletic Journal_ 56 (October 1975): 72–75.

11. Knott, Margaret, and Voss, Dorothy. _Proprioceptive Neuromuscular Facilitation._ 2d ed. New York: Harper & Row, 1968.

12. Holland, George J. "The Physiology of Flexibility: A Review of the Literature." _Kinesiology Review_ (1968), pp. 49–62.

13. Leighton, Jack R. "The Leighton Flexometer and Flexibility Test." _J. Assn. Physical and Mental Rehabilitation_ 20 (May–June 1966): 86.

14. Leighton, Jack R. "On the Significance of Flexibility for Physical Educators." _JOHPER_ 31 (November 1960): 27–28, 70.

15. Neuberger, Tom. "What the Research Quarterly Says About Warm-up." _JOHPER_ 40 (October 1969): 75–77.

16. Roth, Peter, and Benjamin, Ben E. "Warming up vs. Stretching." _Running Times_ 11 (November 1979): 15–20.

17. Shelton, Robert E., Greringer, Leonard O., and Mattes, Aaron L. _Basic Exercises Pre-Conditioning/ Re-Conditioning/Re-Habilitation._ Dubuque, Iowa: Eddie Bowers Publishing Co., 1983.

18. Stewart, Gord, and Faulkner, Bob. _Bend and Stretch: Suppleness and Strength Exercises._ Victoria, B. C., Canada: Fitness Group, 1979.

Warm-Up Exercises
Neck Rotation (5–7)
Overhead Shoulder Stretch (5–12)
Standing Groin Stretch (5–16)
Side Bends (5–14)
Head-to-Knee Stretch (5–23)
Bending Forward Stretch (5–24)
Hip Flexor Stretch (5–21)
Lying Hamstring Stretch (5–26)
Quadriceps Stretch (5–32)
Calf Stretch (5–34)

Note: Other stretches may be included or substituted to satisfy individual needs.

FIGURE 5.1 *Stretching Program for Pre- and Post-Aerobic Training*

Warm-Up Exercises
Relaxation Stretch (5–6)
Shoulder and Side Stretch (5–9)
Shoulder and Chest Stretch (5–10)
Head-to-Knee Stretch (5–23)
Bending Forward Stretch (5–24)
The Yogi Stretch (5–17)
Standing Groin Stretch (5–16)
Sitting Groin Stretch (5–19)
Hamstring Stretch (5–31)
Calf Stretch (5–34)

Note: Other stretches may be included or substituted to satisfy individual needs.

FIGURE 5.2 *Stretching Program for Pre- and Post-Anaerobic Training*

Warm-Up Exercises
Relaxtion Stretch (5–6)
Neck Rotation (5–7)
Assisted Shoulder and Chest Stretch (5–11)
Standing Groin Stretch (5–16)
Head-to-Knee Stretch (5–23)
The Yogi Stretch (5–17)
Foot-to-Hand Stretch (5–25)
Quadricep Stretch (5–32)

Note: Other optional stretches may be included or substituted to satisfy individual needs.

FIGURE 5.3 *Stretching Program for Pre- and Post-Strength Training*

Warm-Up Exercises
Relaxation Stretch (5–6)
Neck Rotation (5–7)
Overhead Shoulder Stretch (5–12)
Shoulder and Chest Stretch (5–9)
Head-to-Knee Stretch (5–23)
Bending Forward Stretch (5–24)
The Yogi Stretch (5–17)
Standing Groin Stretch (5–16)
Hamstring Stretch (5–26)
Sitting and/or Lying Groin Stretch (5–19, 5–20)
Calf Stretch (5–34)
Ankle Stretch (5–37)
Quadricep Stretch (5–32)
Relaxation Stretch or Hang on Bar

Note: Other stretches may be included or substituted to satisfy individual needs.

FIGURE 5.4 *Stretching Program for Pre- and Post-Football Practice*

Warm-Up Exercises
Relaxation Stretch (5–6)
Neck Rotation (5–7)
Overhead Shoulder Stretch (5–12)
Trunk Rotation (5–15)
Sitting Groin Stretch (5–19)
Back Stretcher (5–27)
Low-Back Stretch (5–28)
Hamstring Stretch (5–31)
Lying Hamstring Stretch (5–26)
Calf Stretch (5–34)
Heel Cord Stretch (5–36)
Ankle Stretcher (5–37)
Hang on Bar

Note: Other stretches may be included or substituted to satisfy individual needs.

FIGURE 5.5 *Stretching Program for Pre- or Post-Basketball Practice*

6

Conditioning for Injury Prevention and Rehabilitation

When athletic trainers and sports medicine physicians discuss athletic injuries, they invariably emphasize the importance of preventive measures. Foremost among preventive recommendations has been the warning that many sports injuries are the result of inadequate physical conditioning.[12] Until recently there was very little documentation of the conventional wisdom that preconditioning is essential to prevent or reduce the chance of sports injuries.

Although overuse training can lead to injury, as detailed in Chapter 8, it is often the result of a previously inactive athlete moving too rapidly into intense training or competition.[6] Many sports medicine experts not only emphasize the importance of conditioning but also recommend specific exercises related to the particular type of joint stress the athlete will undergo. Olson[10] described the effectiveness of off-season conditioning as a deterrent to injury in high school football. Burkett's[3] classic work on hamstring injuries highlighted the importance of muscle strength balance. He found that a strength imbalance as small as ten percent led to a seventy percent chance of injury to the *weaker* hamstring. Other studies[1, 5] have also confirmed the effectiveness of reducing athletic injuries by preconditioning.

PREVENTION OF ATHLETIC INJURIES

Many precautions can be taken to prevent athletic injuries, including the use of quality equipment and facilities, proper medical care and athletic training, and physical and psychological readiness for the sport. It has been recognized for some time that a large percentage of athletic injuries are caused by inadequate physical conditioning. The conditioning program should include the proper balance of aerobic and anaerobic training, flexibility, strength, and agility to meet the demands of the sport.

Conditioning for aerobic power has been described elsewhere as important in enabling the athlete to practice longer and harder with less fatigue and less susceptibility to injury. In most circumstances when the fatigue is a prevalent factor in injury, it is the general endurance of the athlete (aerobic power) that is found lacking. The athlete should be conditioned by gradual increases in the intensity of either practice or play. Anaerobic conditioning must precede vigorous anaerobic performance on the part of the athlete. Oftentimes injury is the result of a more forceful muscular contraction than the athlete is prepared to make. The proper mechanics of a new skill should be learned before the athlete attempts the skill under full speed or maximum force conditions.

Sufficient flexibility is necessary to reduce the potential of muscle, tendon, and ligament injuries. Strains, pulls, stretches, and tears may result from a lack of flexibility. Both general stretches for the entire body and special stretching exercises for specific movements of the sport are recommended. Athletes vary in the amount of stretching necessary to prepare them for competition and conditioning. Some have a greater tendency for muscle cramps, strains, and pulls while others may require additional stretching in particular areas of the body. Techniques for static stretching are discussed in Chapter 5 and are considered by the authors to be an integral part of any conditioning program.

The strength training programs offered in the text include strength exercises designed to reduce the potential of injury to the athlete. Some strength exercises are included to protect specific areas of the body susceptible to injury because of the nature of the particular sport. Some athletes will require strength exercises designed to reduce a personal weakness or a muscular imbalance, i.e., one muscle of a paired group being weaker than the other. There is evidence that muscular imbalance may be the cause of one of the most nagging sports injuries, the hamstring pull. As mentioned earlier, specificity also applies to preventive conditioning. If muscular endurance, speed, and range of motion are required of the sport, then the conditioning program must match those requirements. The human body (muscles and joints) is subjected to tremendous stresses and forces during athletic performance. If these stresses and forces are the result of high speed movement on the part of the limbs, then the muscles and joints should be prepared by high speed conditioning.

Preventive conditioning is well worth the time and effort. Any athlete or coach who has had to deal with injuries will agree that prevention is preferable to rehabilitation.

REHABILITATION

Extreme caution is urged in retraining an athlete after injury. Several steps should be taken before rehabilitation is attempted.

1. When an injury first occurs, it should be reported immediately to the team trainer—or to the coach if no trainer is available. This should be done regardless of how minor the injury may appear. If the injury is obviously serious or if it persists, a doctor should be consulted.
2. If there is a period of latency from the regular athletic activity, the physician should be consulted before activity or reconditioning is undertaken.
3. The advice and directions of the physician should be followed precisely. The physician may indicate medical implications that are not apparent to the trainer, coach, or athlete. Un-

fortunately, the supply of good sports physicians is not abundant. Sometimes the athletic trainer may be more familiar with sports injuries than the physician, who may also not be familiar with the demands of the sport. The physician, coach, trainer, and athlete should work together to help rehabilitate the athlete. The physician should be expected to prescribe exercises after serious injury.

Several questions should be considered before initiating a rehabilitation program: What type or combination of exercises should be done, e.g., walking, stretching, running, swimming, weight training, or agility exercises? How intense should each type of exercise be? What is the purpose of each exercise prescribed by the physician? How can the athlete tell whether he or she is doing too much of any type of exercise? What is the expected length of the period of retraining before recovery is complete? How can the athlete tell when he or she is fully recovered?

It may be necessary to have someone assist the athlete in the early stages of rehabilitation. That individual may help the athlete perform the exercises, or even manually guide the athlete through the range of motion to reduce the effort on an injured limb. Rehabilitation of injuries must obviously be very individualized, but there are general guidelines to follow.

Guidelines for Reconditioning

1. The reconditioning program or exercises prescribed by the physician should be carefully followed.
2. Begin conditioning slowly and easily. Increase speed and intensity very gradually.
3. Be certain that movements are done smoothly, avoiding jerky or stressful movements of the joints.
4. Some discomfort is to be expected when performing exercises, especially as the amount or intensity increases. Sharp pain or increasing discomfort is the signal that the exercise must be discontinued or modified.
5. General conditioning or conditioning of specific parts of the body should be maintained, whenever feasible, during the period of latency.
6. Low resistance and high repetition (fifteen to twenty-five reps) is usually the rule for rehabilitative exercises.
7. Rehabilitation should not result in the over-

development of one limb. It may be necessary to train the opposing muscle group or limb. If an injured limb is very heavily retrained, muscular imbalance may result.

Rehabilitative exercises may be done daily or even several times per day. In some circumstances greater rest may be required and rehabilitative sessions may be held less often. The concept of active rehabilitation is widely used in medicine and can hasten the recovery of the athlete. Impatience is probably the greatest danger to the athlete during the rehabilitative period.

INJURY PREVENTION AND REHABILITATION EXERCISES

The following are stretching, strength, and agility exercises that are particularly valuable in injury prevention and/or rehabilitation. Other exercises not described here can be found in either Chapter 4 or Chapter 5.

Foot, Ankle, and Calf Exercises

Calf Stretcher (See Chapter 5)
Toe Raises (See Chapter 4)

Ankle Rotation. This exercise is done by placing a towel (folded lengthwise) on the floor in front of a chair or bench. A weight (about ten pounds) is placed on the end of the towel. In the sitting position, the athlete then pulls the towel across by placing his foot on the towel and rotating the ankle. He then lifts the foot and reaches over and pulls more towel across. This can be done ten or fifteen times with each foot. To strengthen the antagonistic muscles, the movement may be done in the opposite direction.

Golf Ball Pick-up with Toes. In this exercise a golf ball is lifted by the toes. It can be held for as long as possible, then placed back on the floor and repeated with the other foot. After the toes have exercised holding the ball, they can be stretched or spread while the other foot flexes.

Dorsiflexion of Foot. This movement, which involves the muscles in the front of the calf, the foot, and the ankle, can be strengthened by having the athlete or a partner provide the resistance by hand. Static stretching can be done in each direction

before and/or after the strength exercise. The resistance should be steady and should allow smooth movement through the entire range of motion.

Another method of strengthening this area involves hanging a weight from the end of the toe. A strap eighteen inches long and a high table on which to sit are necessary to perform this exercise. The strap is tied to the ankle with the end hanging over the toe. A weight (five to fifteen pounds) is then tied to the strap. It is helpful if the strap is taped to the shoe so that it will not slip off the toe. This method takes more time than the manual method, and for that reason is usually used for rehabilitation rather than as a preventive measure. In such cases, the dorsiflexion of the anke should be accompanied by alternating inversion and eversion of the foot. This can be done every other set or every other rep. This movement may also be strengthened using a standard leg extension, leg curl machine.

PHOTO 6.1 *Dorsiflexion of Foot*

PHOTO 6.2 *Dorsiflexion of Foot (with Weight)*

Ankle Strengthener and Stretcher. This exercise is done to prevent ankle sprains. Some arc-shaped footing six to ten inches deep and approximately 3½' X 3½' is needed.

Jumping on either the convex or concave surface creates inversion and eversion of the feet, strengthening the feet and ankles. Approximately the same number of repetitions should be done on each type of surface so that balanced muscular development is ensured.

Knee and Thigh

Toe Raises (See Chapter 4)

Leg Extension. This exercise is done on a "quad" or leg-extension machine by taking the resistance through a range of motion from where the knee is flexed to where it is fully extended.

PHOTO 6.3   *Leg Extension*

Leg Curl (See Chapter 4)
Half Squat (See Chapter 4)

Lateral and/or Diagonal Leg Motion (with pulley or ankle weight).   After the ankle is attached to a pulley, the leg, with the knee completely extended, is adducted or abducted so that resistance is applied laterally to the knee. See Photo 6.4.

Single Leg Lifts.   These are done as the initial rehabilitation exercise of the knee, especially when complete mobility cannot be or has not been restored.

Double Leg Lifts (See Chapter 5)
Head to Knees (See Chapter 5)
Wide Straddle Seat (See Chapter 5)
"Good Morning" Exercise (See Chapter 4)
Hyperextension (See Chapter 4)
Half Squat (See Chapter 4)
Sit-Ups (See Chapter 4)
Single Leg Lifts (See Chapter 5)
High Knee Lift (See Chapter 4)

Lateral Leg Lift.   This exercise is performed by lying on the side and raising one leg as high as possible, by abducting the hip then lowering the leg slowly. This can be done without resistance as a stretch or with ankle weights. A weighted boot or a floor pulley can be attached to the ankle.

Hip Extension (with pulley or weighted boot).   This exercise is done in the prone position by attaching a high pulley to the ankle. The range of motion is basically the same as the Single Leg Lift except that the resistance is in the opposite direction, thus exercising the muscles of the hips and lower back.

Hip Circumduction (with angle weight or weighted boot).   This movement is done by moving the foot through a circular pattern while abducting and adducting the hip.

Head-to-Knee Stretch (See Chapter 5)
Yogi (See Chapter 5)
Foot-to-Hand Stretch (See Chapter 5)
Wide Straddle Seat (See Chapter 5)
Stiff-legged Dead Lift Stretch (See Chapter 4)

Hand and Wrist

Wrist Curl (See Chapter 4)
Wrist Roller (See Chapter 4)
Reverse Curl (See Chapter 4)
Squeezing Rubber Ball

Wrist Flexion and Extension (with dumbbell). This exercise is done with a light dumbbell by flexing and extending the wrist so that the largest and smallest joint angles are alternately opposed to the thumb and fifth finger.

Wrist Rotation (or supination and pronation with dumbbell). This exercise is done by simply rotating the wrist back and forth while holding a dumbbell.

Finger and Hand Flexion and Extension. This is done as a stretch by simply alternating the spreading of the fingers (complete extension) and clenching of the fist.

PHOTO 6.4   *Lateral and/or Diagonal Leg Motion*

Elbow

Curl (with dumbbell or pulley for rehabilitation) (See Chapter 4)

Reverse Curl (with dumbbell or pulley for rehabilitation) (See Chapter 4)

Tricep Extension (lying, sitting, or standing with dumbbell) (See Chapter 4)

Arm Circles. These are done with the elbows extended and the arms straight out to the sides, making small circles in either or both directions. They may be done with no weight or with a light (five to fifteen pound) dumbbell.

Forearm Circles. These are done by holding the elbow at the side, contacting the body. The hand is then moved in a circular motion. This should be done in both directions. A dumbbell is usually used but the exercise may be done without weight when necessary.

Bar Dips (See Chapter 4). For rehabilitative purposes these can be done between two benches or chairs, with the legs supported on the floor.

Bench Press (See Chapter 4)

Lateral Raises. These are done in the standing position by elevating (abducting) the shoulders. The arms which are held straight out to the sides are moved to a position directly overhead. See Photo 6.6.

Shoulder Exercises

Bar Dips (See Chapter 4). For rehabilitative purposes these can be done between two benches or chairs, with the legs supported.

Bent Arm Laterals (See Chapter 4)

Incline Flys. These are simply Bent Arm Laterals done on an inclined bench. The upper chest and shoulders are strengthened. See Photo 6.7.

Bent Arm Pullovers (See Chapter 4)
Military Press (See Chapter 4)
Lat Pulls (See Chapter 4)
Bench Press (See Chapter 4)

Straight Arm Hanging. This is done by simply hanging from a chinning bar. It can be done for from one to sixty seconds.

PHOTO 6.5 *Arm Circles*

PHOTO 6.6   *Lateral Raises*

Neck

Neck Extension (See Chapter 4)
Neck Flexion (See Chapter 4)
Neck Rotation (See Chapter 4)
Shoulder Shrug (See Chapter 4)

Isometric and Isotonic Neck Exercises.   Resistance is applied smoothly by a partner. This is a quick

and fairly effective way to warm up or strengthen the neck.

SUMMARY

In this chapter we have discussed the need for preventive conditioning exercises to reduce the potential for injury. Such exercises include aerobic and

PHOTO 6.7 *Incline Flys*

anaerobic conditioning, flexibility, agility, and strength. Basic guidelines for rehabilitation are listed and the role of the physician in rehabilitation is stressed. Preventive and rehabilitative exercises are listed, some of which also appear in Chapters 4 and 5.

REFERENCES

1. Abbot, H. G., Kress, J. B. "Preconditioning in the Prevention of Knee Injuries." *Arch. Med. Rehabil.* 50 (June 1979): 326–333.
2. Arnheim, Daniel D., and Klafs, Carl E. *Workbook in Sports Injury: Prevention and Management.* St. Louis: C. V. Mosby Co., 1977.
3. Burkett, Lee N. "Causative Factors in Hamstring Strains." *Medicine and Science in Sports* 2 (1970): 39–42.
4. Burkett, Lee N. "Cause and Prevention of Hamstring Pulls." *Athletic Journal* 51 (1971): 34.
5. Cahill, B. R., Griffith, E. H. "Effect of Preseason Conditioning Program on the Incidence and Severity of High School Football Knee Injuries. *Am. J. Sports Med.* 6 (July 1978): 180–84.
6. Clement, D. B., Taunton, J. E., Smart, G. W., McNicol, K. L. "A Survey of Overuse Running Injuries." *Phys. Sportsmed.*, 9(5) (May 1981): 47–58.
7. deVries, Herbert A. "Flexibility, an Overlooked but Vital Factor in Sports Conditioning." *Proceedings: International Symposium on the Art and Science of Coaching*, pp. 209–221. Ontario, Canada: F. I. Productions, 1971.
8. Dominquez, M. D.: "Shoulder Pain in Swimmers." *Phys. Sportsmed.* 8(7) (July 1980): 37–48.
9. Klafs, Carl E., and Arneheim, Daniel D. *Modern Principles of Athletic Training*, 5th ed. St. Louis: C. V. Mosby Co., 1981.
10. Olson, C. C. "The Spokane Study of High School Football Injuries." *Phys. Sportsmed.* 7(12) (December 1979): 75–80.
11. Ryan, Allan J. "The Role of Training and Conditioning in the Prevention of Athletic Injuries." *Health and Fitness in the Modern World*, pp. 302–307. Chicago: Athletic Institute, 1961.
12. *Sports Injuries: An Aid to Prevention and Treatment.* American College of Sports Medicine, American Orthopaedic Society, and The U.S. Tennis Association. 1983.

7

Sports Nutrition

Efforts to improve athletic performance through manipulation of the diet date back to antiquity. The practice of having athletes consume large amounts of meat (protein) to build muscle tissue probably originated with the Greeks. Unfortunately, many myths and misconceptions have haunted nutritional practices over the years. Although nutrition has grown in stature as a science in this country, nutritionists must constantly remind the public as well as athletes and coaches of the basic principles of nutrition. Coaches and athletes often lose sight of the basic function of foods in an effort to uncover exotic diets or combinations of foods that are reputed to improve athletic performance. The first portion of this chapter will serve as a reminder of the basic function of nutrition.

Throughout the world nutrition plays a major role in the maintenance of health. The relationship between malnutrition and the various deficiency diseases is most evident in developing countries or in areas of the world that lack sufficient food.[2] An abundance of food, rather than a shortage, is generally characteristic of the United States. Some nutritionists and medical scientists claim that the major nutrition-related health problems in this country involve overconsumption of calories and poor food selection despite the general abundance. Public knowledge about good nutrition is growing significantly, but many myths and misconceptions about proper nutrition still persist.

GOOD NUTRITION

Nutrition can be defined as the "science of food and its relation to optimal health and performance."[2] It involves nourishing the body properly. This means providing adequate: (1) fuel for energy,

(2) material for building and maintenance, and (3) nutrients for regulating the bodily processes. One of the major functions of nutrition is to keep calorie input and output in balance (energy balance). This concept is particularly important for athletes in training, which involves major increases in energy output. A major chore for most athletes is consuming sufficient calories to maintain energy balance and to *not* lose weight. Details of energy balance for athletes will be discussed later in the chapter. Energy balance assumes not only sufficient fuel for sports activities but also sufficient maintenance materials for bodily tissues.

The digestive system is physiologically responsible for breaking down foods into usable nutrients, leading to good nutrition. The process involves enzymes which are secreted in the small intestine and "break down" food mechanically and chemically. From the small intestine, the broken-down foodstuffs are absorbed into the blood to enter into the metabolic cycle. A detailed description of digestion or the biochemistry of muscular energy is beyond the intended scope of this chapter. Both processes involve a complex series of biochemical steps that are linked together. A simplified description of muscle-energy metabolism can be found in Figure 7.1.

Figure 7.1 illustrates the importance of both carbohydrates (CHO) and fats in supplying energy for sports activities. Protein is *not* a significant energy supply in physical activity. As described in Chapter 3 (Conditioning/AER-AN), the real "fuel" for sports activities at the muscle tissue level is ATP (adenosine triphosphate). ATP is a high-energy phosphate found in the muscle fiber. The foods that we consume are directly involved in the metabolic processes which ultimately enable ATP to "explode" in the muscle tissue and produce contraction. Thus the cookie that the athlete consumes days before the athletic contest eventually

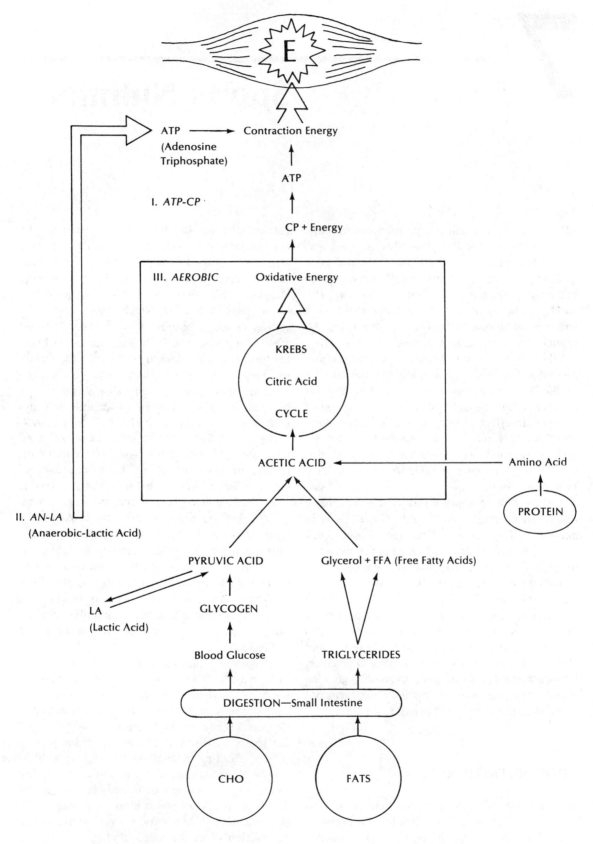

FIGURE 7.1 *Muscle-Energy Metabolism*

is involved in contributing energy for the resupply of ATP to fuel muscle contraction during the sports event.

BASIC NUTRIENTS

There are six classes of basic nutrients: protein, carbohydrates, fat, vitamins, minerals, and water. Carbohydrates, protein, and fat are the most abundant nutrients in our diet and the only ones that supply energy (calories) during sports or work activities. Nutrients are the important chemical substances responsible for nourishing the body properly, i.e., (1) supplying energy, (2) providing building and maintenance materials, and (3) regulating bodily processes.

It is estimated that there are about fifty basic nutrients needed by the human body.[10] Ten of those nutrients are considered to be "leader" nutrients and are described in Figure 7.2. A balanced diet which supplies sufficient amounts of the ten leader nutrients will probably supply enough of the other forty basic nutrients.

Each nutrient has a specific effect that can be fulfilled only by that nutrient. In some instances nutrients must work together as a team in order to produce a desired effect. Nutrients are found in food, but in varying amounts in different foods. All of the nutrients needed for good nutrition for anyone, including athletes, can be obtained by eating a *variety* of different foods. Therefore, it is particularly important to consume a variety of different foods. It is also the reason why nutritionists educate us to consume the "balanced diet."

Carbohydrates

CHO is the most abundant nutrient and is the major source of energy in our diet. The range of calories supplied by CHO in most diets is from 45 to 60 percent. Nutritionists and sports scientists generally agree that athletes as well as nonathletes can benefit from a complex CHO intake on the high end of that range. There is no minimum requirement for CHO, which is primarily an energy nutrient in anaerobic activities. It should be noted, however, that excess intake of CHO is converted to fat and stored in the body. CHO loading is one of the few successful manipulations of diet to influence athletic performance. See Carbohydrate Loading later in this chapter.

The principal kinds of CHO are sugars and starches. Starches are complex forms of sugar which are broken down by digestion into simple sugar such as glucose. It should be noted that both starches and sugars can be broken down into glucose but at a different rate. Complex CHO breaks down more slowly than do simple sugars. In addition, starches usually contain more nutrients and dietary fiber than do simple sugars. The energy yield of CHO is 4.3 calories per gram, which is similar to that of protein. Since two-thirds of the stored glycogen in the body is found in the muscles, it is obviously important for athletes to maintain sufficient muscle glycogen levels.

Protein

Protein must be resupplied daily via essential amino acids (EAA). The range of calories supplied by protein in most diets is from 12 to 20 percent. Because protein is involved in building bodily tissue, including muscle, it has often been assumed that a high protein intake is necessary for athletes. Most Americans on an adequately balanced diet are consuming twice as much protein (100 gm/day) as necessary (46 gm/day). Although it is an extremely important nutrient, protein is frequently overconsumed.

Animal protein is of high quality and a complete source of EAA. Vegetable protein, on the other hand, is incomplete unless combined with some animal protein. This is a very important concept for athletes. A vegetarian diet is usually *not* compatible with intense athletic conditioning and competition unless it is very carefully and scientifically designed.

Fat

Fat is an essential component of the balanced diet; it represents a concentrated form of energy. Fat supplies twice as many calories (9.5/gm) as CHO or protein (4.3/gm). The range of calories supplied by fat in most diets is 25 to 45 percent. For good health fat consumption should be on the lower end of that range, for both athletes and nonathletes.

Because excess fat consumption is often associated with overweight and heart disease, fat is frequently overlooked as a basic and necessary nutrient. Fat is a major fuel in aerobic exercise and

Nutrients for health

Nutrients are chemical substances obtained from foods during digestion. They are needed to regulate body processes and to supply energy.

About 50 nutrients, including water, are needed daily for optimum health. If one obtains the proper amount of the 10 "leader" nutrients in the daily diet, the other 40 or so will likely be consumed in sufficient amounts.

One's diet should include a variety of foods. No single food supplies all the 50 nutrients, and many nutrients must work together.

When a nutrient is added or a nutritional claim is made, nutrition-labeling regulations require listing the 10 leader nutrients on food packages.

Protein

Supplies four calories of energy per gram

Sources: Meat, fish, poultry, dried beans and peas, egg, cheese, milk

Functions: Constitutes part of the structure of every cell. Supports growth and maintains healthy body cells. Constitutes part of enzymes, some hormones and body fluids, and antibodies that increase resistance to infection.

Carbohydrate

Major souce of energy for central nervous system—four calories per gram

Sources: Cereal, corn, potatoes, dried beans, bread, sugar

Functions: Supplies energy so protein can be used for growth and maintenance of body cells. Unrefined products—complex carbohydrates in fruits, vegetables and whole grains—supply fiber for regular elimination. Assists in body's use of fat.

Fat

Supplies nine calories of energy per gram

Sources: Shortening, oil, butter, margarine, salad dressing, sausages

Functions: Constitutes part of the structure of every cell. Supplies essential fatty acids. Provides and carries fat-soluble vitamins (A, D, E and K).

Vitamin A (Retinol)

Sources: Carrots, liver, greens, sweet potatoes, butter, margarine

Functions: Assists formation and maintenance of skin and mucous membranes (such as nasal passages and intestinal tract), increasing resistance to infection. Functions to promote healthy eye tissues and eye adaptation in dim light.

Vitamin C (Ascorbic acid)

Sources: Broccoli, grapefruit, orange, strawberries, papaya, mango

Functions: Forms cementing substances, such as collagen, that hold body together. Strengthens body, hastens healing, increases resistance to infection. Aids body's use of iron.

Calcium

Sources: Milk, yogurt, cheese, sardines and salmon with bones, kale, mustard, collard and turnip greens

Functions: Combines with other minerals to give structure and strength to bones and teeth. Assists in blood clotting. Functions in normal muscle contraction and relaxation and normal nerve transmission.

Niacin

Aids in utilization of energy

Sources: Liver, meat, poultry, fish, peanuts, fortified cereal products

Functions: Functions as part of a coenzyme in fat synthesis, tissue respiration and body's use of carbohydrate. Aids digestion and fosters normal appetite.

FIGURE 7.2

Thiamin (B₁)
Aids in utilization of energy

Sources: Lean pork, nuts, fortified cereal products

Functions: Functions as part of a coenzyme to promote body's use of carbohydrate. Promotes normal appetite. Contributes to normal functioning of nervous system.

Riboflavin (B₂)
Aids in utilization of energy

Sources: Liver, milk, yogurt, cottage cheese

Functions: Functions as part of a coenzyme in production of energy within body cells. Promotes healthy skin and eyes.

Iron
Aids in utilization of energy

Sources: Enriched farina, prune juice, liver, dried beans and peas, red meat

Functions: Combines with protein to form hemoglobin which carries oxygen to cells. Prevents nutritional anemia. Increases resistance to infection. Functions as part of enzymes involved in tissue respiration.

FIGURE 7.2 (Continued)

has other essential functions in the body, as shown in Figure 7.2. A major function is its role in carrying the fat-soluble vitamins. It is also true that many nutritionists and medical scientists recommend a low to moderate intake of saturated fats to reduce the potential of coronary artery disease.

Vitamins

Vitamins do not supply calories (energy); rather, they function as catalysts or action regulators in body metabolism. In that way, their function is not unlike the inorganic elements and hormones that are involved in human metabolism.

There are Recommended Dietary Allowances (RDA) of the various vitamins to prevent vitamin deficiency diseases. Many athletes and nonathletes have consumed excessive amounts (megadoses) of vitamins. This has not proved beneficial to athletic performance or to health in general. Moreover, some excess consumption can be toxic. It is the fat-soluble vitamins which are stored in the tissues of the body that have the potential for excessive buildup and toxicity. The fat-soluble vitamins include vitamins A, D, E, and K. Their sources and functions can be seen in Figure 7.2.

The water-soluble vitamins must be replenished daily. They are not stored in the tissues, and excess consumption is not toxic (but does produce the world's most expensive urine!). The water-soluble vitamins include Vitamin C and the B complex

(Thiamin, Riboflavin, and Niacin). The function of those vitamins and good sources of them are seen in Figure 7.2.

Minerals

Small amounts of essential minerals must be ingested or deficiency diseases can occur. The classic example is iron deficiency, which, it is estimated, affects 15 percent of the population of the United States. Among the most essential mineral nutrients can be found iron, iodine, calcium, phosphorus, sodium, and potassium. Calcium and phosphorus help build strong bones and body structure. Some of the essential minerals are involved in the energy metabolism of sports activities, while others are important in maintaining water balance for the athlete. See Figure 7.2.

Water

Water is frequently overlooked as a basic nutrient. It is, however, the second most important element for sustaining life, overshadowed only by oxygen. The maintenance of water balance is a crucial function of the body and is extremely important for the athlete. Water is responsible for regulating body temperature and dissolving and transporting nutrients and other essentials.

BASIC FOOD GROUPS

In order to ensure that sufficient amounts of the basic nutrients are consumed, the Recommended Dietary Allowances (RDA) were developed and are constantly being restudied and revised.[15] Most of the nutrients and amounts listed on the RDA are not meaningful except to nutritionists and scientists. A simplified guide for athletes and nonathletes is the United States daily food guide, which identifies the four Basic Food Groups (Figure 7.3).

Figure 7.3 lists the number of servings recommended in each of the four Basic Food Groups and what constitutes a serving. By consuming the recommended number of servings daily, the athlete or nonathlete is assured of meeting the RDA, with few exceptions. Each food group makes specific nutrient contributions. Foods from all of the groups work together to supply energy and

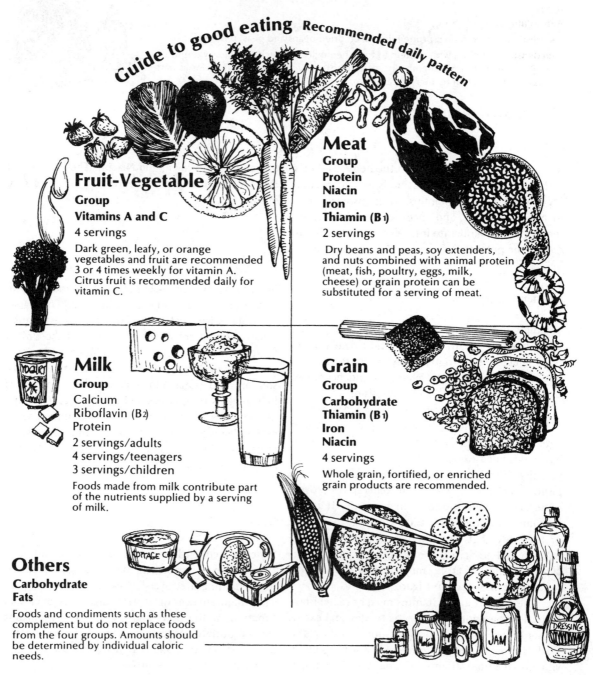

Guide to good eating Recommended daily pattern

Fruit-Vegetable
Group
Vitamins A and C

4 servings

Dark green, leafy, or orange vegetables and fruit are recommended 3 or 4 times weekly for vitamin A. Citrus fruit is recommended daily for vitamin C.

Meat
Group
Protein
Niacin
Iron
Thiamin (B₁)

2 servings

Dry beans and peas, soy extenders, and nuts combined with animal protein (meat, fish, poultry, eggs, milk, cheese) or grain protein can be substituted for a serving of meat.

Milk
Group
Calcium
Riboflavin (B₂)
Protein

2 servings/adults
4 servings/teenagers
3 servings/children

Foods made from milk contribute part of the nutrients supplied by a serving of milk.

Grain
Group
Carbohydrate
Thiamin (B₁)
Iron
Niacin

4 servings

Whole grain, fortified, or enriched grain products are recommended.

Others
Carbohydrate
Fats

Foods and condiments such as these complement but do not replace foods from the four groups. Amounts should be determined by individual caloric needs.

FIGURE 7.3   *Basic Food Groups*

nutrients for good health and growth. The intake can be easily adjusted to meet the needs of special groups such as growing children or teen-agers. It is important to note that persons of all ages and both sexes require food selections from each of the four groups daily.

NUTRITION AND THE ATHLETE

It is often difficult for coaches and athletes to believe that some magic manipulation of the diet will not produce better physical performance. Studies of dietary supplements have repeatedly confirmed that improved performance will not occur as a result of extra intake of vitamins, proteins, or other supplements. Rogozkin[12] states that the major concerns for sports nutrition include: (1) providing adequate energy supplies (calories), (2) maintaining a balanced diet, (3) choosing adequate forms of nutrition, and (4) dealing with individual needs (weight gain or loss) and likes and dislikes.

The authors do not imply that good nutrition is a simple process. Detailed study of the nutrition of athletes reveals a very complex process influenced by many variables. Muscle glycogen levels are important in many sports performances and there are ways of increasing the resting levels. Many females, including female athletes in heavy training, are susceptible to iron deficiencies. As a result of medical screening, iron supplements are recommended for many female athletes in heavy training. An important aspect of sports nutrition is an understanding of the basic information that has preceded this section. In the next section the special aspects of nutrition for athletes will be discussed.

Energy Balance

The relationship between caloric expenditure (output) and caloric consumption (intake) represents energy balance. If intake and output are balanced, body weight will remain constant. If caloric consumption *exceeds* physical activity, the excess intake is stored as fat and the individual gains weight. This is a major cause of obesity in our society. If the physical activity *exceeds* the caloric intake, the individual loses weight by diminishing fat storage.

The amount of calories required per day for a "moderately active" college student is estimated to be 15 calories times the body in pounds. Thus a 125-pound female would require 1,875 calories per day to maintain energy balance (15 × 125 = 1,875), while a 175-pound male would require 2,625 calories. A wide range of daily caloric consumption can exist for individuals of similar "moderately active" levels. The range might extend from 1,500 calories for a 100-pound person to 3,375 calories for a 225-pound individual.

The athlete in training and competition is more than "moderately active." An athlete can easily burn 1,000 to 1,500 additional calories in a lengthy vigorous workout. A more realistic caloric consumption per pound for athletes could be 20, resulting in a daily consumption of 2,500 calories for the 125-pound female athlete and 3,500 calories for the 175-pound male. The caloric consumption for many large, highly trained athletes has been found to be in the range of 4,000 to 6,000 calories per day. This is not an astounding intake when one considers the size of the athletes and the number of workouts per day. Football players who undergo two or three-a-day workouts consume 4,000 to 6,000 calories daily without gaining weight because of the tremendous energy expenditure. Many may actually lose weight under such regimens despite a generous training table. Vigorous activity raises metabolism for many hours after the exercise is over. This additional burning of calories is *in addition to* the calories burned during the exercise.

Besides the body weight of the athlete, the duration and intensity of the sports activity should be considered in estimating the caloric consumption for maintaining energy balance. The caloric cost of several sports activities is listed in Figure 7.4.

Age will also have a bearing on the caloric consumption of young athletes. Boys and girls aged 10 to 12 years will require approximately 30 calories per pound daily, while junior high and high school athletes (aged 14 to 18) will require approximately 23 calories per pound of body weight daily.[9] As the authors have previously stated, college athletes, usually between the ages of 18 and 22, will require approximately 20 calories per pound daily. As a result, an athletic 12-year-old boy may consume as many calories daily as a college-age female athlete (75 lbs. × 30 = 2,250 calories *versus* 110 lbs. × 20 = 2,200 calories).

If the athlete must lose weight, it is recommended for good nutrition that caloric intake not fall below certain base levels. Those levels are 1,600 calories per day for female athletes and

♀		♂
125 lbs.	Activity	178 lbs.
700-1000	Running (7-12 mph)	1000-1400
—	Wrestling	900
550	Swimming (Crawl)	600-750
550	Jogging	750
500	Racquetball	750
450	Soccer	650
350-500	Basketball	500-700
350-500	Tennis	500-700
—	Football	600
300-500	Volleyball	400-700
250-300	Softball/Baseball	325-425
200-275	Golf	300-400

FIGURE 7.4   Caloric Cost of Sports Activities
(Calorie Per Hour)

2,000 for male athletes.[7] Sufficient base levels are necessary to maintain adequate nutrient intake for good nutrition. It is unlikely that many athletes would need to lose weight, as we shall see below.

Body Composition

The need to lose weight is not usually a problem for athletes since being over-fat is usually associated with below-normal activity levels. Excess fat stored in the body is also detrimental to physical performance, and it is unlikely that an athlete could achieve successful performance in an over-fat state.

At this point it is appropriate to distinguish between overweight and obesity. *Overweight* refers to body weight exceeding the standard height/weight charts. *Obesity* refers to excess body fat above the recommended levels. It is not uncommon for athletes, both male and female, to be overweight according to the height/weight charts, but not be obese. As a matter of fact, many such athletes are actually less fat than average individuals.

Body composition is made up of : (1) Lean Body Weight (LBW), which is composed of muscles, bones, and connective tissue, and (2) fat weight. The percentage of body weight in fat is a far more accurate determinant of the athlete's fatness than is the weight alone when compared to the height/weight charts. If we consider two athletes of the same height and weight (150 pounds), one may be considerably fatter than the other. At 150 pounds, one athlete may have 15 pounds of fat, or 10 percent of body weight in fat.

The other athlete may have 30 pounds of fat, or 20 percent of fat weight. From an athletic performance standpoint, the second athlete is over-fat but not, perhaps, overweight according to the height/weight charts.

Occasionally both male and female athletes are overweight according to the height/weight charts. For example, a 225-pound football player may exceed the weight chart by 25 or 30 pounds according to height. If he is heavily boned and muscled, which is very likely, he may be only 10 to 12 percent fat, which is below average for his age and sex. Coaches and athletes need to be aware that the percentage of body fat is far more important in determining an ideal weight than height/weight charts and the scale. Sometimes coaches and athletes expect additional weight loss when the athlete is already extremely lean. This may result in weight loss from the muscle tissue (LBW) and may have a negative effect on performance. Some standards for percentage of body fat are listed in Figure 7.5. Athletes are generally very lean, compared to the college-age populations. (See Figure 7.5.)

Measurement of body fat. How is body fat measured? The most accurate (but time-consuming) technique is underwater weighing. The technique is designed to measure body density and is usually done in medical clinics or university laboratories. To simplify the concept, the reader should recall that the body composition includes LBW and fat. Since muscle and bone are heavier by volume than fat, the individual with *less* fat will have a higher

Females		Males
<17%	Lean—"Athletic"	<9%
18-19%	Below Average	10-11%
20-23%	Good—Average	12-15%
24-30%	Above Average	16-20%
>31%	Obese	>21%

ATHLETES

Females		Males
12-14%	Runners	4-6%
	Gymnasts	6-8%
16-20%	Basketball	
	Football—Backs	6-9%
	Football—Linemen	12-14%
23%	"Non-Athletes"	15%

FIGURE 7.5   Standard for % Body Fat
College Age Males, Females, and Athletes

body density. Fat does not "weigh" in water; rather, it floats. Let us consider again an individual who weighs 150 pounds (dry) on the scale. When weighed underwater, the individual may "lose" 15 pounds of body weight which can be assumed to be fat. That 15 pounds represents 10 percent of the total body weight when dry—hence, 10 percent body fat. The technique is actually more complex than described here because we must also consider the air trapped in the lungs, which makes the individual more buoyant and less dense. (See Figure 7.6.)

A simple and less time-consuming technique for estimating body fat involves the use of skinfold calipers. The skinfold technique involves measuring a "pinch" of subcutaneous fat at several anatomical sites. While the skinfold is not as accurate for estimating body fat as is underwater weighing, it is reasonably accurate to use in clinical and athletic settings. Correlations between skin-

fold techniques are high enough for predictions ($r = .90$) if the skinfolds are taken accurately by an experienced individual. Formulas have been devised to estimate percentage of body fat from several (one to six) skinfold site measurements. The formulas for skinfold estimates of body fat are very age- and sex-specific, i.e., they are designed to be used *only* on persons of the same sex and in a narrow age range. Specific formulas have been devised for athletes in training, and they can be very accurate if proper techniques are employed. Figure 7.7 illustrates the skinfold technique.

Lean body weight (LBW). Among the many beneficial effects of exercise training on the body is a decrease in stored body fat and an increase in LBW, primarily muscle tissue. This effect is added to the self-selection process which discourages over-fat individuals from remaining in sport while encouraging those with a higher muscle mass and less

$$\% \text{ Body Fat} = \frac{\text{Weight (dry)} - \text{LBW}}{\text{Weight (dry)}} \times 100$$

FIGURE 7.6 *Measurement of Body Fat (Underwater Weighing)*

FIGURE 7.7 *Measurement of Body Fat (Skinfold Technique)*

body fat. Some athletes may actually desire to gain weight for added body mass. From the previous discussion it is evident that it is most desirable for weight gain in athletes to be primarily in LBW or muscle tissue. It can be accomplished by increasing caloric intake while concentrating on muscle tissue building exercise (weight training). Aerobic exercise will tend to counter these efforts since it consumes calories (primarily fat) over long periods of time.

Carbohydrate Loading

It was previously recommended that the ideal distribution of nutrients in a balanced diet for athletes, as well as others, be comprised of total calories: 55 to 60 percent carbohydrates, 25 to 30 percent fat, and 10 to 15 percent protein. Carbohydrate represents the most important fuel source during exercise. It is the sole energy source during anaerobic activity and is also a significant source, along with fat, during aerobic activity.

Fat cannot be adequately utilized during aerobic activity without sufficient stored glycogen.

Glycogen is an extremely important fuel source during sports performance. About two-thirds of the glycogen in the body is stored in the muscles; one-third is stored in the liver. For most sports activities, stored glycogen is far more than sufficient to maintain the ATP cycle. This is especially true of anaerobic performances which last for only brief moments and are not carried on long enough to seriously deplete muscle glycogen. Many vigorous team sports which combine both aerobic and anaerobic metabolism, however, will gradually reduce muscle glycogen. This is particularly true over a period of time when several games are played in a few days. Generally it takes 24 to 48 hours to replace muscle glycogen, even on a 60 percent CHO diet.[3]

The main exception to the concept that dietary manipulation cannot significantly alter performance is the employment of CHO loading. CHO loading is effective *only* in athletic situations that call for sustained high energy expenditure over a long period of time, e.g., the marathon. While team sports may gradually erode some muscle glycogen over several days, the endurance athlete (such as the marathoner) can face rapid depletion of muscle glycogen in just a few hours. The CHO loading technique has proved to be an effective way to increase stored muscle glycogen and thus to enhance performance.[4]

There are several techniques that have proved to increase stored muscle glycogen. The most simple method involves increasing carbohydrate intake for several days prior to an endurance event while simultaneously reducing physical training. The most effective technique, however, involves a week-long plan of diet and exercise. As the competitor approaches the final week before the endurance event, the process is begun. About seven days before the event, the athlete engages in a final exhausting and glycogen-depleting workout. This results in a muscle glycogen level that falls below normal. For several days the athlete continues to work out (not as vigorously) and consumes a *low* carbohydrate diet. This results in additional lowering of muscle glycogen levels. In the last several days prior to the event the athlete consumes a very high CHO diet and ceases work, or reduces it to a minimum. A significant rebound effect occurs, and muscle glycogen may exceed the normal resting level by nearly three times, just prior to the event. This effect can mean a significant difference in the athlete's performance.

A few words of *caution* are in order about CHO loading. First, it has a very limited use in sports, namely, for intense endurance events such as the marathon. Even when used by endurance athletes, it should be employed infrequently. It is not a nutritionally sound diet to be used weekly because it becomes very unbalanced with high fat and protein consumption followed by high CHO intake. In addition, some athletes do not tolerate high carbohydrate diets well. Elevated blood glucose from the high carbohydrate intake may result in excessive insulin secretion, which results in abnormally lowered blood glucose. This over-reaction by insulin is also known as hypoglycemia. It is generally recommended that the athlete experiment with CHO loading long before a major event, to determine if the brief unbalanced dietary routine is well tolerated.

It has been noted earlier that athletes consume many more calories daily than do normally active individuals. Much of the additional intake of calories is in the form of carbohydrate. This is beneficial for two reasons: (1) less fat is consumed proportionally, which is beneficial from the health standpoint; and (2) CHO is the major source of energy fuel for the body.

Protein Intake

Much of the mystique associated with diet and sport involves protein. Since muscle tissue is largely protein, athletes from antiquity to today have assumed that muscle tissue must constantly be replenished. Protein is not a source of muscle energy, as was thought in the past, and it should constitute only 10 to 15 percent of caloric intake. Protein is used as tissue-building material, and some athletic diets have been as high as 20 percent of calories in protein. It is often a surprise to most individuals, especially to coaches and athletes, that protein can constitute such a small proportion of the diet. Significant increases in the protein component of the diet do not enhance physical performance, nor do they increase muscle tissue.

Most Americans consume far more protein than is necessary for good health or optimum performance. The recommended protein intake for moderately active individuals is approximately one gram per kilogram of body weight (1 gm/kg).[10] A 165-pound (75 kg) athlete on a 3,000-calorie-per-day diet would receive 75 to 112 grams of protein if the diet were 10 to 15 percent protein. The requirement for that athlete would be 75 grams of protein per day. First, the recommended allowances are set high; then most individuals overconsume protein, so the error is usually on the plus side. As the activity level of the athlete increases, the caloric intake increases and keeps pace with any additional demand. The 253-pound (115 kg) football player on a 5,000-calorie-per-day intake will receive 138 to 187 grams of protein if the diet is only 10 to 15 percent protein.

When excessive amounts of protein are taken in, since they are not required for food, they are excreted by the body. Some excess protein can also be converted to fat, but the major portion of it will be excreted by the kidneys. It joins overdoses of water-soluble vitamins to produce that expensive urine mentioned earlier. Even if the protein requirements of athletes were doubled, the demand could still easily be met by most American diets.

Water Balance

As mentioned earlier, water is rarely recognized as an essential nutrient by most persons. Adequate water intake is very critical for athletes. Perhaps nothing produces so detrimental an effect on performance as rapidly as does dehydration. Most of the life-threatening situations associated with physical activity and sport involve dehydration. Exercise in high heat and humidity conditions can lead to rapid water loss and can require special attention. Studies of exercise and water intake in hot environments have repeatedly demonstrated that voluntary intake of water *does not* keep up with water loss. Athletes replenished only about two-thirds of the loss. Even forced water intake during exercise in heat fails to balance water loss completely. Water balance means that water in all forms of liquid or foods must constantly balance water lost from the body by urination, perspiration, and other sources. Since it appears difficult for the body to maintain water balance during and immediately after exercise, additional water is taken in for many hours after exercise. In some cases, water balance may not be re-established for 24 hours.

Under moderately active conditions, approximately one liter of water is required for each 1,000 calories of food consumed daily.[7] Thus athletes on 3,000-5,000-calorie-a-day intake should consume at least 3 to 5 liters of water. When high heat or humidity adds to the metabolic heat of exercise, *additional* amounts of water are required.

Fortunately coaches have abandoned withholding of water during practice and performance. That practice only hastens fatigue. Most coaches and athletes now recognize the need to maintain water intake during prolonged periods of heavy exercise. Perhaps the major question remaining involves how to schedule water intake to best bring about water balance. A few principles of sound water intake are as follows:

1. Ensure that the athlete is well hydrated during the weeks and days prior to the event. In the hours before activity the athlete should take in additional fluid, especially in hot weather.
2. During practice or an event it is best to schedule water intake in small amounts every 15 minutes or so. Since water is continually being lost during exercise, this procedure is preferable to attempting to "load up" before and after practice or a game.
3. Athletic drinks can be important in replenishing glucose and potassium. It should be noted, however, that water intake should be the first priority, and that water loss will begin to affect performance before electrolyte loss. In addition, the high concentration of glucose in athletic drinks will pull additional water from the tissues to balance higher concentrations of blood glucose. The solution to this problem for many endurance athletes is to dilute the athletic drink with water, or merely restrict fluid intake to water only.

Dehydration is a serious problem and it can proceed rapidly under certain conditions (high heat and humidity, heavy exercise, and insufficient water intake). The combination of those conditions can be deadly. Nearly every year dehydration problems cause one or more deaths in sports, usually in late summer as high school and college football players practice under the conditions listed above. Another group of athletes who habitually flirt with serious dehydration problems are wrestlers. Medical and sports medicine groups have consistently warned the wrestling community about the dangers of "making weight" through voluntary dehydration.[16] They have suggested that a standard weight be established on the athlete during the off- or pre-season, and that weight loss be controlled and limited on the basis of that weight.

Dehydration can become a serious problem for wrestlers. As a group, wrestlers, like many other athletes, are very lean with the exception of those in the upper weight categories. There are limits to the amount of fat weight loss that can occur to athletes who are already below 10 percent body fat, or in some cases at or below 5 percent fat. No one knows the minimum limit to body fat before additional loss becomes detrimental to health. It is known, however, that as fat stores are seriously diminished, the body resists additional loss of fat. Some observers have identified 5 percent as "essential" fat. This means that at very low body fat levels, additional weight loss is accomplished primarily by water (possible dehydration) and LBW (muscle tissue) loss. Both of these losses are detrimental to physical performance. A rapid loss of only one percent of body weight begins to affect performance, and at 3 to 5 percent, the performance will be seriously affected.

Perhaps the most reasonable approach for wrestlers is to establish the standard weight during the off-season, as was earlier suggested, and to monitor body composition carefully. As the wrestler reaches 5 percent body fat, no additional weight loss should be permitted, since it is likely to be at the cost of body water and muscle tissue. Remember that a 10- or 20-pound weight loss has a much greater effect on a 120-pound wrestler than on a 200-pound wrestler. A higher percentage of body water and muscle tissue will be lost by the smaller wrestler.

The Pre-Game Meal

Much of the mysticism associated with the pre-game meal is also diminishing. The old habit of high protein (steak and eggs) intake before the contest has proved not beneficial for two reasons: (1) protein is not a major source of energy fuel, and (2) high protein intake may cause additional water loss during digestion and metabolism. The preferred, and recommended, pre-game meal should be relatively high in carbohydrate. This will require additional water intake to assist in glycogen storage. Meals high in complex carbohydrate will usually be easy to digest, and CHO will be reduced to simple sugars more slowly. Since glycogen utilization comes from muscle stores during most sports events, it does little good to load the body with simple sugars just prior to activity. This procedure results primarily in elevating blood glucose. Such a practice may be beneficial, however—even necessary—during prolonged activities, since muscle glycogen and blood glucose can both be depleted. The marathoner, again, is the best example.

A few simple principles are suggested for the pre-game meal:

1. Have the athlete eat at least two to three hours before activity. Although complete digestion will not occur during that time, most food will have left the stomach.
2. A meal high in complex carbohydrates (starches) such as spaghetti or pancakes is preferred. The likes and dislikes of the athlete should be considered also, and a choice of several dishes high in CHO is suggested.
3. The "liquid meal" is preferred by many coaches and athletes because of its nutritional balance and ease of digestion. Many athletes, including professionals, are too anxious before a contest to eat normally. The liquid meal has the additional advantage of adding fluid at a time when it is very much needed. If a liquid meal is not selected, it is imperative to remind the athlete of the importance of consuming water with the pre-game meal.

SUMMARY

It is hoped that this discussion of sports nutrition has illustrated the importance of consuming a well-balanced diet of sufficient calories to maintain good health as well as sports performance. Perhaps the greatest concern for coaches and athletic trainers is that teen-age athletes may be prone to poor nutritional habits regardless of family income. Both boys and girls are likely to resort to "junk food" during a busy schedule period. Although coaches frequently voice a need to be more knowledgeable about nutrition in general, they usually do not establish diet as high priority in the preparation of the athlete. It is strongly recommended that they, as well as athletic trainers, take an active part in disseminating accurate nutrition information to athletes. Where appropriate and feasible, they should also assist in the selection of food for the athlete.

REFERENCES

1. Astrand, Per-Olaf, and Rodahl, Kaare. *Textbook of Work Physiology*. 2d ed. New York: McGraw-Hill, 1977.
2. Briggs, George M., and Calloway, Doris H. *Bogert's Nutrition and Physical Fitness*. 10th ed. Philadelphia: W. B. Saunders Co., 1979.
3. Costill, David L. "Sports Nutrition: The Role of Carbohydrates." *Nutrition News* 41 (February 1978): 1, 4.
4. Fox, Edward L. *Sports Physiology*. 2d ed. Philadelphia: W. B. Saunders Co., 1984.
5. Fox, Edward L., and Mathews, Donald K. *The Physiological Basis of Physical Education and Athletics*. 3d ed. Philadelphia: Saunders College, 1981.
6. Katch, Frank I., and McArdle, William D. *Nutrition, Weight Control and Exercise*. Boston: Houghton Mifflin Co., 1977.
7. Lapidus, Jayne. "Basic Nutrition for Sports Participants." *Osteopathic Annals* 7 (October 1979): 18–21.
8. "Nutrition and Physical Fitness." *Journal of the American Dietetic Association* 76 (1980): 437–443.
9. *Nutrition for Athletes*. Reston, VA: AAHPERD, 1971.
10. *Nutrition Source Book*. Rosemont, IL: National Dairy Council, 1978.
11. Palumbo, John D., and Blackburn, George L. "Human Protein Requirements." *Contemporary Nutrition* 5 (January 1980): 1–2.
12. Parizkova, Jana, and Rogozkin, V. A., eds. *Nutrition, Physical Fitness, and Health*. Baltimore: University Park Press, 1978.
13. Serfass, Robert C. "Nutrition for the Athlete Update, 1982." *Contemporary Nutrition* 7 (April 1982): 1–2.
14. *Sports Nutrition*. Department of Nutrition and Food Service, Tucson: University of Arizona, 1982.
15. "Toward a National Nutrition Policy." *Nutrition News* 9 (December 1980): 1–2.
16. "Weight Loss in Wrestlers." ACSM Position Stand. *Medicine and Science in Sports* 8 (Summer 1976): xi-xiii.
17. Young, D. R. *Physical Performance Fitness and Diet*. Springfield, IL: Charles C Thomas, 1977.

PART II

CONDITIONING PROGRAMS FOR SPORTS

This section of the book deals with the application of conditioning programs to specific sports. The introductory material (Chapter 8) offers practical suggestions to the coach for employing conditioning programs off-season, pre-season, and within the regular practice session (in-season). The remaining chapters offer specialized programs in football, soccer, basketball, hockey, volley ball, wrestling, baseball, softball, swimming, track and field, and individual sports (archery, golf, gymnastics, and tennis).

General conditioning, stretching, and strengthening of basic muscle groups may be beneficial to nearly any sports performer. There are distinct differences, however, in the way various factors such as strength, speed, or endurance contribute to the performance of different sports skills. The objective of the conditioning programs for the various sports covered in this volume is to match the training techniques as specifically as possible to the demands of the sports.

8

The Conditioning Program: Putting It All Together

Guidelines and principles for using conditioning programs in the off-season, pre-season, and in-season are discussed in this chapter. Ways of implementing a year-round conditioning program are developed for the coach and athlete. In Chapter 3 we discussed specific techniques for developing aerobic and anaerobic conditioning, in Chapter 4 we discussed specific techniques for developing strength for sports, and in Chapter 5 we discussed techniques for increasing flexibility in sports. Armed with the basic information developed in those chapters, and with the principles suggested for putting the program all together, the coach or athlete should be better able to use the programs designed for specific sports in subsequent chapters.

YEAR-ROUND CONDITIONING

The concept of year-round conditioning may appear alarming to some coaches and athletes. Younger athletes especially should be given an opportunity to develop skills and playing ability in a variety of sports before concentrating on one sport or one position. In Youth Sports Leagues the major objective is fun, and conditioning should not become a year-round chore. Many experienced athletes and even professionals object to the concept of conditioning year round. For the athlete who has reached the level of specialization, how-

ever, year-round conditioning is essential in order to remain competitive.

Year-round conditioning is a logical step aimed at improving performance, maintaining sports conditioning, and preventing injuries. The authors have already discussed at length the contributions conditioning can make to improving performance and preventing injuries. All of the training effects described so far are reversible, thus training at various levels must be maintained year round.[6, 16]

DE-CONDITIONING

While most research conducted in the conditioning area looks at training effects, there is some information on de-training or de-conditioning. Most athletes and coaches are familiar with the de-conditioning effect that takes place during periods of no training. It is most evident after the off-season when an athlete has not maintained sports conditioning. The professional football player often waits until pre-season camp before announcing a retirement. That announcement frequently comes after several days of trying to get an "out-of-shape" body back into playing condition. In most instances it cannot be done, and probably the difficulty could have been avoided with some low-intensity off-season work.

Sports conditioning, which is often achieved

after many weeks and months of concentrated effort and hard work, can be lost very rapidly. Every training effect previously discussed can be rapidly lost. Aerobic power is lost rapidly while strength decreases more slowly. Even within two weeks there can be a significant reduction in work capacity. Depending upon the initial level of condition, the loss of work capacity can drop from 50 to 100 percent in three to eight months.[12]

Total rest is not essential for the de-conditioning effect to take place. Since training effects and sports conditioning are specific, discontinuance of one aspect of training can result in a loss of power in that system. Kroll[8] found a loss in throwing power in a collegiate baseball team that discontinued weight training *during* the season. Of greater interest is that a second baseball team *maintained* a reduced-strength training program in season and lost no throwing power. Clarke[3] reports that once strength has been built to a plateau, it can be maintained with as few as one training session per week. Coleman[4] found that major league baseball players actually increased strength and reduced body fat with approximately two strength training sessions per week. Also of importance, the degree of muscular symmetry was greater than that of teammates who did not maintain a strength program in season. All of these changes occurred without a loss of flexibility.

Athletes in a predominantly anaerobic sport can also lose AER power if AER training is not maintained in season. Hickson and Rosenhoetter[7] found that AER power could be maintained with as little as two conditioning sessions per week. This format followed a strenuous six-day-a-week training routine for ten weeks. The two-day-a-week maintenance program held AER power at a constant level for fifteen weeks. This is a very important concept for coaches and athletes– namely, that maintenance programs either off-season, and especially in season, do not require as much time as does the developmental phase of training.

OFF-SEASON CONDITIONING

Many professional athletes and high-level performers recognize the necessity to maintain physical condition during the off-season. Maintenance of aerobic and anaerobic condition and strength for sports reduces the chore of pre-season conditioning for both the coach and the athlete. For professional athletes, maintaining sports condi-

tioning can oftentimes mean a prolonged athletic career. For the young and developing athlete, the off-season conditioning program may be a particularly important time for developing strength and sports fitness.

During the off-season coaches and athletes will usually reduce the concentration of time spent on developing sports skills and strategy. This enables the athlete to place greater concentration on physical conditioning in terms of time and effort. In the school setting the coach will often recommend an extensive physical conditioning program for athletes during the summer months. Varying concentrations should be made on aerobic, anaerobic, strength conditioning, and flexibility during the off-season.

Aerobic Conditioning

In Chapters 2 and 3 we outline the basic reasons for the development of good aerobic conditioning for most team sports. The off-season period is an ideal time to concentrate on aerobic conditioning for athletes. Time is available for the continuous type of training described in Chapter 3. Continuous aerobic conditioning, such as running two to three miles at least three times a week, is an effective means of developing a good aerobic conditioning base for the athlete. A GOAL can be established during the off-season conditioning program, such as being able to run 2.0 miles in fifteen minutes or less as a minimum requirement for entering pre-season conditioning for all athletes. The intensity of off-season AER conditioning should be low (65-75 percent) with emphasis on continuous work (LSD).

Anaerobic Conditioning

Anaerobic conditioning does not receive as much emphasis during the off-season as does aerobic conditioning. There are several reasons for this situation. For sports that rely heavily on aerobic and anaerobic conditioning, such as track and field and swimming, the intensity of training gradually increases from the off-season to the pre-season to the in-season period. Athletes and coaches in these sports prefer to have a peaking of athletic performance toward the latter stages of the sport season.

Anaerobic conditioning is very intense, both

physiologically and psychologically. Anaerobic interval training produces a great deal of work during the training session, as described in Chapter 3, but it also leaves the athlete with a high level of fatigue. During in-season training coaches and athletes will avoid repeated days of intense anaerobic interval training because of the accumulated fatigue.

Real problems of psychological fatigue occur when intense anaerobic training is carried on for months on end. This form of training requires a great deal of persistence and motivation on the part of the athlete. Inhibition can be built up in the athlete if it is carried on year round. Therefore, anaerobic training receives little attention during the off-season.

Strength Training

Since the athlete is not engaged in regular athletic competition during the off-season, he or she can afford to undertake a more intensive strength program. The intensity of the force of contraction of the muscle determines the amount of strength the muscle can develop. Heavier weights are thus used during the off-season, resulting in a reduction in the speed of contraction. The athlete should nevertheless concentrate on making the contraction as explosive as possible. Although the slower speed is not immediately advantageous to performing high-speed athletic movements, the overall increase in strength is desirable at this time and serves as a basis for strength development similar to the "basis" role of aerobic training prior to anaerobic training. Later (pre-season and in-season), speed of muscle contraction will be increased to match more specifically the speed of the sports skill. Strength training in the off-season thus focuses on slower speed movements and fewer repetitions than most sports usually require.

The number of repetitions of each exercise to be done in the off-season will be less than the number done in-season. Even for high endurance sports, this number will be below ten.

The year-round strength program should entail a cohesive plan aimed at: (1) developing maximum strength off-season; (2) adjusting the strength levels to match the muscular endurance, range of motion, and speed of the sport pre-season; and (3) maintaining the strength with those specific characteristics in the off-season. The general rule is that fewer repetitions will be used in the off-

season. It should also be emphasized that many different systems of training containing a wide variation of sets and reps have been shown to be effective.

Flexibility

Flexibility training "knows" no season. Flexibility must be maintained year round and does not require, at any time, intense effort from the athlete. Special remedial exercises are sometimes used during the off-season but the basic aims and programs of flexibility should be consistent throughout the year. The athlete should continue to work on either the development or the maintenance of flexibility throughout the year.

PRE-SEASON CONDITIONING

The objectives of a year-round conditioning program are to develop and maintain aerobic conditioning and strength during the off-season, increase the intensity of aerobic conditioning during the pre-season, and peak and maintain aerobic, anaerobic, and strength conditioning during the in-season period. (See Figure 8.1) If off-season programs are used properly, pre-season conditioning can be designed to bring the athlete to a peak of condition in the briefest possible time. Coaches and athletes are well aware of the time pressures during the pre-season period to develop physical skills and strategy, and also physical conditioning. During the pre-season coaches often must resort to prolonged practice sessions or multiple sessions during the practice days.

Aerobic Conditioning

Aerobic intervals can be used during the pre-season conditioning period to develop peak aerobic condition. An example of aerobic intervals would be:

	Distance	% Max	Rest
RUN	½ mi.	80% +	3–5 min.

	Reps	Times per Week
	4–6 times	3

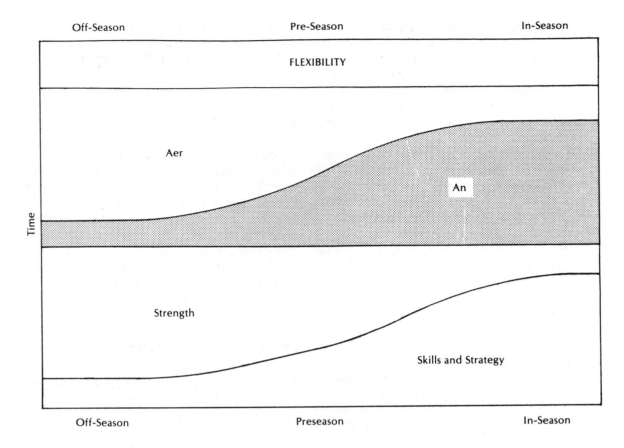

FIGURE 8.1   *Year-Round Conditioning*

Aerobic intervals as compared with continuous aerobic work, will increase the intensity of the aerobic conditioning and also begin to incorporate some anaerobic conditioning. Since the aerobic work is not as intense as anaerobic conditioning, it is recommended that the aerobic portion of the pre-season practice session be done at the beginning of the session and be incorporated as part of the warm-up. If all four conditioning systems will be involved in a single training session or circuit, it is generally recommended that flexibility and aerobic training precede strength training, with anaerobic training concluding the session. (See Figure 8.2)

Anaerobic Conditioning

Interval training will be utilized to develop anaerobic capacity, as described in Chapter 3. An example would be. Sprinting fifty to one hundred yards, all-out; rest period, five to fifteen seconds; five to twenty reps, five times per week. Anaerobic conditioning should come at the latter portion of

(a)   *Treadmill Test of Maximal Aerobic Power (VO$_2$ max)*

(b)   *Bicycle Ergometer Test of VO$_2$ max*

Warm-up and Stretching	5–10 mins.
Aerobic Conditioning	15–20 mins.
Strength Training	15–45 mins.
Anaerobic Conditioning	15 mins.
Stretching	5 mins.
	30–90 mins.

FIGURE 8.2   *The Conditioning Session*

the practice session during the pre-season program because of the fatigue built up during intense interval training.

Strength Training

The main goal of the pre-season strength program is to prepare the athlete to meet the strength demands of the sport. Strength must be adjusted to be usable at the specific speed, muscular endurance, and through the exact range of motion of the sport. Special concentration is also given at this time to the areas of the body most vulnerable to injury.

Special high-speed equipment can be used at this time, if it is available. The circuit training technique is recommended by the authors because of the potential time savings and combining of aerobic, anaerobic, and strength conditioning. For more specific information about the adjustments in the strength program pre-season, see Chapter 4.

IN-SEASON CONDITIONING

It is the authors' contention that far too many coaches and athletes abandon serious physical conditioning during the in-season period. The reasons voiced are usually lack of time, the claim that conditioning is unnecessary during the season, and the difficulties of arranging a conditioning program in terms of facilities and equipment. The authors maintain that the rationale for year-round conditioning including in-season work, is well established in Part I of this book. Physical condition and strength increases are *reversible*. The athlete who trains seriously and diligently during the pre-season period faces the prospect that a certain amount of de-conditioning may take place during the season. This is particularly true for sports that are not physically demanding, and for athletes who do not receive a great deal of playing time during the season.

The problems of time and equipment are real and are not minimized by the authors. We contend, however, that it is both necessary and possible to maintain aerobic conditioning and strength during the in-season period. Coaches and athletes probably find more time for anaerobic conditioning during the in-season period than the other two conditioning systems, perhaps because it generally requires less time.

Aerobic Conditioning

Aerobic conditioning can be maintained for most sports with as little as two or three training sessions per week of from five to fifteen minutes. Obviously, this minimum time period will not suffice for highly aerobic sports, but should maintain base aerobic conditioning for most team sports. A combination warm-up run and aerobic conditioning period prior to practice will meet the requirements set forth for maintaining aerobic conditioning During the season AER conditioning generally should be of higher intensity (75-85 percent) and less time (intervals) than the off-season period.

Anaerobic Conditioning

Anaerobic conditioning can be maintained by essentially the same interval training techniques used in the preconditioning period. The intensity and duration of the interval training should be determined by the anaerobic demands of the sport; i.e., the more anaerobic sports will require anaerobic training of greater intensity during the in-season period.

Strength Training

The main goals of in-season strength training are to maintain the strength level demanded of the sport and to help prevent injuries. Like aerobic conditioning, strength and power can be maintained by far less work than is required to attain peak levels of strength and power. For most team sports, one or two strength training sessions per week will be sufficient to maintain strength.

The same number of repetitions are usually followed during the in-season program as in the pre-season period, although the amount of resistance may be reduced slightly. Concentration is still focused on speed of movement, maintenance of muscular endurance, and exact range of motion. Short sessions will produce sufficient work to maintain usable strength. Athletes who are capable of increasing resistance during this period should do so gradually, taking care not to sacrifice speed or endurance.

To aid in injury prevention, the areas of the body most subject to injury should be given special attention. (See Chapter 6.) Maintaining strength in those muscle groups will reduce the risk of muscle injury.

Within-Practice Conditioning

One technique of aerobic and anaerobic conditioning often overlooked by coaches and athletes is within-practice conditioning. This term simply suggests that aerobic and anaerobic overload can occur during skills practice or in actual game practice in several ways. Coaches and athletes should be alert to take advantage of conditioning opportunities within the skills practice session. In football, for example, when plays are run continuously without a huddle, as is done in the two-minute drills, there is overload on the anaerobic system. In basketball, repeated fast break drills also produce an overload on the anaerobic system. In both examples the athlete is practicing the skills involved in the sport, but he is also producing higher levels of conditioning in the anaerobic system.

Scrimmage sessions in basketball may be held continuously without break for substitutions, free throws, or other time-out. This is an excellent example of aerobic conditioning taking place within the practice session. Continuous play in volleyball can produce similar aerobic conditioning results.

Opportunities for aerobic and anaerobic conditioning in less physically demanding sports will obviously be limited. This is the major rationale for supplementary conditioning, as outlined in Part I of this book. The coach or athlete, however, who does not take advantage of opportunities to condition during the practice session is not really making the best use of the time available for full development of the athlete.

Sometimes the coach must make decisions as to when certain conditioning areas should be stressed during the practice session. As mentioned earlier, there is a recommended sequence to follow for conditioning activities whether they stand alone in the off-season or are incorporated within the practice. It is not recommended that strength training be conducted on the same day as intense anaerobic work. The general sequence of activities is illustrated in Figure 8.2. Flexibility exercises will always precede and conclude practice or conditioning sessions. Aerobic work should come early in the session since it is low in intensity and can also serve to prepare the athlete for more intense conditioning. Skills practice or strategy work should follow (if appropriate). Either strength training or anaerobic conditioning should occur in the latter part of the session because of the intensity and residual fatigue. (See Figure 8.2.)

Circuit Training

Circuit training has many advantages for total conditioning, and they are outlined in detail in Chapter 3. Because of these advantages (leading to aerobic, anaerobic, and strength conditioning) the authors recommend circuit training as an ideal way of putting all conditioning together during the in-season program. A circuit specific to the individual sport involved can be easily utilized by the athlete or coach. Such a circuit can include muscular endurance, flexibility, and agility exercises as needed by the specific sport. Circuits designed for a number of specific sports are outlined in subsequent chapters.

OVERTRAINING

Staleness or overtraining is a problem that worries both coaches and athletes. It has a physiological basis when associated with overconditioning, and it has a psychological basis when associated with excess skills practice. Staleness is more than imaginary on the part of an athlete.

Psychologists employ a term that describes the kind of staleness affecting the athlete from overpractice of skills. *Reactive inhibition* means that excessive amounts of practice which have already occurred are affecting the performance at the present time. By repeating a skill over and over, the athlete builds up an inhibition toward repeating the skill again. If we were to observe an athlete practicing under forced conditions over a long period, performance would ultimately begin to deteriorate. The combination of both fatigue and the inhibition toward repeating the performance would result in decreased performance. It is not inferred that fatigue alone is the cause of inhibition. When staleness builds up to this point, the only means of reducing it is to rest or discontinue practice for a time. A few classic examples of athletes who became victims of the Staleness Syndrome in the 1970s and 1980s include Dave Cowens of the NBA, and both Chris Evert Lloyd and Bjorn Borg in professional tennis.

The more effective means of dealing with the problem is to prevent it, by not making practice so continuous and so repetitious that it results in staleness. Rest periods or a change of activity are the best means the coach can use to avoid staleness. Most coaches are well aware of this concept and organize practice with frequent changes of activity.

There can be a physiological staleness resulting from excess conditioning in the practice of highly physical sports. Astrand[2] reminds us that high-level competition requires overload to increase physiological capacities, which means an almost endless cycle of increasing training intensity. This is a good argument to vary sports conditioning and especially to alternate days or periods of high-intensity training with days or periods of low-intensity training. Prokop[11] long ago proposed that there may be a limit to the body's capacity to sustain and adapt to high-intensity training periods. After the initial stress of increased intensity, the body will adapt to conditioning, but if overstressed continually, a declining adaptation will occur within a period ranging from five weeks to three months. Most athletes will show symptoms of overtraining (when it occurs) at approximately six to eight weeks. The symptoms of overstress or overtraining are more than subjective, and the coach and athlete should be alert to their appearance.

The physical symptoms of overstress on the body may be very similar regardless of the nature of the stress. Selye[14] reminds us that overstress results in nonspecific responses, i.e., the same stress symptom may result from very different stressors. Physical manifestations of stress may be a problem for most individuals but they can be insurmountable for the athlete. The athlete relies on, and comes to expect, a good physical response from a well-conditioned body. When overtraining symptoms occur, the results can be devastating for the athlete, both physically and mentally.

With overtraining, some or all of the overstress symptoms may be felt.[10] The muscles may feel stiff and sore, with discomfort in the muscle, joints, or tendons. The athlete sometimes complains of "heavy legs." A frequent symptom involves loss of appetite and body weight. There may be headache, fatigue, and sluggishness; sometimes lymph node swelling and gastrointestinal or stomach disorders. The athlete's physical performance typically declines and he or she may appear nervous, depressed, or unable to relax. The athlete may exhibit loss of interest not only in sports performance, but also a decline in school or other work.

There may be a fine line between optimum or "peak" training and overtraining. No certain method of measuring or anticipating overtraining exists, but some efforts have been made to identify physiological correlates. Many athletes record their resting heart rate (HR) before getting out of bed in the morning. If the HR is eight to ten beats above average, the athlete either lowers the training intensity that day or rests entirely if other symptoms are present (cold or flu). Some swimming coaches have used the same sub-max effort to begin each workout and have recorded HR after the standard work load. If it is above normal, the athlete is instructed to train less intensely that day. The East Germans have even used LA levels as well as HR response to determine the individual variance in response to a standard work load each day. If the LA (Lactic Acid) level is up, the work intensity is reduced. Blood counts have also been used in elite athletes as a measurement of training stress.

In addition to avoiding the results of overtraining (declining performance), efforts to identify overstress are also designed to avoid injury. The rate of injury can be expected to increase with overtraining and indeed some sports injuries are called "overuse" syndromes. Some long-time coaches, especially in track and swimming, maintain that more athletes fail to perform to expectation because of overtraining than from undertraining.

Since there is a lack of clearly effective, yet simple tests to measure potential overtraining, the coach or athlete can best prevent overstress by following several principles.

1. The year-round training routine is designed to prevent a loss of sports conditioning and also to alternate periods of low intensity (off-season), high intensity (pre-season), and maintenance (in-season).

2. High-intensity training should not be continued for long periods. Within two or three months most athletes will encounter a period of declining adaptation and declining performance.

3. An ideal schedule involves alternating days of high or low intensity. If this is not possible, then two or three days of high intensity should be followed by a similar period of low intensity work.

MEASUREMENT OF SPORTS CONDITIONING

A logical question for coaches and athletes is how to measure sports conditioning for aerobic, anaerobic, or strength development. If conditioning is to become a year-round process, then the coach or athlete must have some means of evaluating the progress of the conditioning program. Elsewhere the authors have referred to the establishment of goals to be met at the beginning of the pre-season conditioning period. Any time an athlete begins a conditioning program, it is essential to establish the existing aerobic, and anaerobic, or strength status. Periodic testing then enables the coach or athlete to determine the effectiveness of the conditioning program.

There are no widely used or widely accepted tests of athletic power. Much of the testing of aerobic power or muscular strength has been restricted to performance laboratories. Sophisticated tests requiring extensive equipment have been conducted on athletes in many laboratories, but only a small portion of coaches and athletes have access to such facilities.

Some techniques and field tests could be used effectively to estimate aerobic power, anaerobic power, or strength. The authors have included tests or techniques for each of those areas in the Appendix. Perhaps one of the simplest ways of measuring progress in sports conditioning is to record daily or weekly performance in each of the three areas on recording charts, such as the ones listed in the Appendix.

Aerobic Power

The most accurate test of aerobic power is a maximum treadmill, bicycle ergometer, or bench-step test during which oxygen consumption is monitored. (See Figure 8.3) A variety of tests that involve running, either for time or distance, can very easily be used by the coach or athlete.[1, 5] Such field tests usually estimate aerobic power from distance run in a given time, or from the time it takes to run a specified distance. The authors recommend the use of field running tests to measure aerobic power, as such tests do not require unusual equipment or facilities. Aerobic power field running tests are listed in the Appendix.

Anaerobic Power

Anaerobic power has been the least tested element of sports conditioning. Margaria et al.[9] have devised a simple test of anaerobic power that requires only steps and a stopwatch. The test is described in the Appendix.

Strength

Sophisticated tests of strength can use dynamometers, tensiometers, or isokinetic recording devices. Perhaps the most universally used technique for measuring strength in specific muscle groups is an all-out effort (1RM). That technique can be incorporated periodically on the strength recording sheet that appears in the Appendix.

SUMMARY

In this chapter we have offered suggestions for developing a year-round conditioning program, including off-season, pre-season, and in-season programs. The emphasis on aerobic, anaerobic, or strength conditioning will vary from one part of the season to another. Flexibility training remains constant throughout the year. The authors particularly underscore the need for coaches and athletes to take advantage of conditioning opportunities during the in-season period. A circuit training program is recommended as an excellent technique for developing total conditioning year round and especially during the in-season program. All of the training effects from sports conditioning are reversible and underscore the need to maintain some training out of season. Overtraining is also a potential that should not be ignored by coach or athlete.

REFERENCES

1. *AAHPER Youth Test Manual*, rev. ed. Washington, D.C.: American Alliance for Health, Physical Education, and Recreation, 1976.
2. Astrand, Per Olof, and Rodahl, Kaare, *Textbook of Work Physiology*. 2d ed. New York: McGraw-Hill, 1977.
3. Clarke, David H. "Adaptations in Strength and Muscular Endurance Resulting from Exercise." *Exercise & Sport Sciences Reviews*, vol. 1, 73–102. New York: Academic Press, 1973.
4. Coleman, Eugene A. "In-Season Strength Training in Major League Baseball Players." *The Physician and Sportsmedicine* 10 (1982): 125–126, 129–32.
5. Cooper, Kenneth H. *The Aerobics Way*. New York: M. Evans, 1977.
6. Fox, Edward L. *Sports Physiology*. 2d ed. Philadelphia: W. B. Saunders Co. 1984.
7. Hickson, Robert C., and Rosenkoetter, Maureen A. "Reduced Training Frequencies and Maintenance of

a. Treadmill Test of Maximal Aerobic Power (VO$_2$max)

b. Bicycle Ergometer Test of VO$_2$max

FIGURE 8.3 *Lab Tests of Aerobic Power*

Increased Aerobic Power." *Medicine & Science in Sports and Exercise* 13 (1981): 13–16.

8. Kroll, William A. "The Effects of an In-Season Weight Training Program Upon the Throwing Power of Junior College Baseball Players." Master's thesis, Arizona State University, 1973.

9. Margaria, Rudolf et al. "Measurement of Muscular Power (Anaerobic) in Man." *Journal of Applied Physiology* 21 (1966): 1662–1664.

10. Mirkin, Gabe, and Hoffman, Marshall. *The Sportsmedicine Book*, Boston: Little, Brown, 1978.

11. Prokop, L. "Adrenals and Sport." *Journal of Sports Medicine and Physical Fitness* 3 (1963): 115–121.

12. Pollack, Michael L. et al., *Health and Fitness Through Physical Activity*. New York: John Wiley & Sons, 1978.

13. Wells, Christine L. "Physiological Principles of Training for Maximal Performance." *Arizona JOHPERD* 23 (Fall 1979): 2–7.

14. Selye, Hans. *Stress Without Distress*. New York: Signet, 1974.

15. Stone, William J. "A Pre-Conditioning Program for Team Sports." *Arizona Prep*, 4 (May 1974): 18–20.

16. Stone, William J. "Sports Conditioning." *Osteopathic Annals* 9 (October 1981): 12–15.

9

Football

In this chapter we include aerobic and anaerobic conditioning programs and strength-building programs for football. In order to make the most effective use of the programs offered here, the reader is referred to Chapter 3 for the basis of aerobic and anaerobic training programs, to Chapter 4 for the basis of strength programs, to Chapter 5 for the basis of warm-up and stretching programs, and to Chapter 8 for the most efficient means of incorporating those objectives into a single workout. The programs are offered as off-season, pre-season, and in-season programs at three levels. The three levels include junior high school, senior high school, and college level training programs. The reader is also referred to sample recording charts offered in the Appendix. These charts will facilitate the measurement of progress that the athlete makes on the training program and will also indicate the athlete's standing in regard to training goals.

Football could be described as the "perfect" *anaerobic* game. It requires a maximum of *anaerobic power*. Speed, strength, acceleration, and agility are the basic elements of the game and thus requirements of the athletes who play the game. There is significant evidence that faster, stronger, and more powerful athletes are at a real advantage in football and that those factors can best be developed by specific conditioning[2]. The typical play in football may last three, five, or eight seconds. Occasionally a longer play may last up to fifteen seconds, but this is rare. Football is the epitome of Stage I (ATP–CP) energy metabolism. If all of the time involved in such action is added together, it has been determined that the ball is in play only eight to twelve minutes in the typical sixty-minute game. The remainder of the time is taken up with picking oneself off the turf, walking back to the huddle, listening to the play, and returning to the line-of-scrimmage in preparation for the next burst of energy. A recent Super Bowl was analyzed for "action" and it tallied only twelve minutes. In the NFL most pass plays allow only 3.0 seconds for blocking.

Recovery from all-out bursts of activity requires good *aerobic* capacity. Increasing the general endurance will enable the football player to perform longer with less fatigue. Repeated bouts of maximum effort, such as occur in football, require general endurance as well as local muscular endurance. Football players often fail to see the need for aerobic capacity in a highly anaerobic sport. Repeated bouts of anaerobic effort result in an accumulation of lactic acid. During the approximately 20 to 25-second rest interval between plays, the player shifts to aerobic metabolism and recovery begins. Full recovery is not possible in that time frame, but greater aerobic capacity results in a higher percentage of recovery. While the conditioning to improve football *performance* is primarily short-burst maximum sprinting, aerobic work is also included although its contribution is primarily for *recovery*.

Football is ideally suited to *strength* programs designed to enhance speed, power, acceleration, and agility. The action is "explosive" and the strength training should match the explosive characteristic of the game. Similar to the aerobic basis prior to intense anaerobic training, slower speed, high-strength training will precede the pre-season and in-season emphasis on high-speed "explosive" training. The concepts reviewed here are discussed in more detail in Chapters 3, 4, 5, and 8.

Football is one of the most complex of team games. Not only is there a variety of positions to be played, but players reflect a number of different body types fulfilling very different roles.[1] Because of the complexity of the game and the team, the conditioning program needs to be well organized in order to meet the demands placed on various players. At the professional level, the Dallas Cowboys of the NFL have solved the problem by computerizing their conditioning program.[5] This solves not only various role differences in conditioning but also allows an individualized approach. Most football programs do not have a conditioning coach and a computer available to them. Some conditioning programs divide the football team into four or five groups, while others maintain that all players should follow the same basic program.[3] The authors were successful in developing a year-round conditioning program at Arizona State University by dividing the team into two primary groups, linemen and backs.[4] Significant improvement was found in strength, power, percent body fat, and endurance, in a four-month period. More important, the gains were maintained during the season without interruption of the practice sessions.

JUNIOR HIGH, HIGH SCHOOL, AND COLLEGE FOOTBALL

Junior High School

Athletes in junior high school usually fall in a range of physical development from prepubescent to postpubescent. No other competitive sports age group offers such a wide range of physical development and potential for athletic injury. This presents an unusual challenge to the athlete or coach to select a training regimen that will match the needs of the individual and reduce the potential for injury. Conditioning needs may be met through after-school programs or within the physical education class. A few guidelines are offered for the training of junior high footballers.

Training sessions should be limited to two or three per week for junior high athletes. Intense anaerobic training should not become such a heavy burden that young athletes become mentally and physically "turned off." Since football requires a high level of tolerance to pain and discomfort, the young athlete should be *gradually* conditioned to undergo vigorous training and play.

Weight training at this level will not be as highly specialized as later, when it becomes directed toward improving performance at a single position. It should be directed primarily toward developing total body strength and enhancing fundamental

athletic skills such as running, jumping, and throwing. Combination programs that include aerobic, anaerobic, and strength training are recommended.

High School

Most high school athletes have completed the adolescent growth spurt and have gravitated toward a particular sport and position. A few youngsters will be multisport athletes. In the day of age-group (Pop Warner, Little League) programs, specialization can occur earlier and certainly the high school athlete will be more specialized than the junior high athlete. He is also prepared to undergo more intensive supplementary training.

The athlete and coach should develop conditioning programs that can be conducted in the off-season (summer). For the novice strength trainer, the coach should include instructions with conditioning programs or refer the athlete to an experienced strength coach. High school is a good time for football players with serious ambitions about athletic careers to become familiar with year-round conditioning.

Young athletes must be cautious in the early stages of weight training and avoid the temptation to lift as much weight as possible (1RM). Heavy squats, to the parallel position (upper leg) or lower, *should not* be attempted by young athletes. The long-term goals of strength training for athletics should be emphasized rather than short-term efforts at maximum strength. Progress can be very motivational for the high school or junior high athlete if records are maintained as suggested by examples in the Appendix. Six to eight weeks of conditioning can produce gains significant enough to impress the most eager young athlete.

Collegiate Football

Like his professional counterparts, the collegiate football player is usually the epitome of specialization. Special-position strength programs are offered later in this chapter to accommodate the special positions. The principles involved in training are essentially the same, however, as for younger athletes. Collegiate football programs pioneered the conditioning approaches that are commonly used at the high school and junior high school level.

There is likely to be a great diversity of

equipment available at the collegiate level. High-powered athletic programs at major universities may have a wide range of strength building equipment at hand. Some collegiate football players have limited experience with weight training or off-season conditioning. Most institutions have "strength coaches" whose major responsibility will be to develop conditioning programs for athletes. The conditioning of the collegiate player is essentially the same as for the professional.

OFF-SEASON

The major objectives of the off-season program are the development of maximum *strength* and *aerobic power*. Both of these objectives require time and, as mentioned earlier, time is available during the off-season to concentrate on these two objectives. Greater aerobic capacity will enable the football player to recover from the repeated anaerobic bursts of activity that characterize football. Greater general endurance means the ability to practice or play longer and harder without becoming fatigued as readily as those who do not train aerobically!

The strength conditioning during the off-season will focus on high resistance, low repetition work. The speed of contraction will be slower than

pre-season and in-season training because of the greater resistance. The off-season is the ideal time for the football player to concentrate on the two objectives (strength and aerobic power) that are less specific to the game than the pre-season and in-season objectives (anaerobic and explosive power).

A circuit training program is frequently designed for off-season conditioning. An entire program can be completed in approximately one hour if a standard "universal type" gym is available. If other types of gym machines and/or free weights are available, a circuit can also be designed.

In designing a circuit, it is desirable that the muscle groups being used be varied so that two consecutive stations do not use the same muscle group as the main movers. If barbells are available, the Clean and Squat movements should be included. The Clean is imitative of the fundamental explosive football movement necessary to deliver a rising blow.

Additional exercises can be done to improve throwing power if a wall pulley, Apollo, Mini-Gym, or some such other pulley device is available. When training with wall pulleys to improve throwing, the exact range of movement should be followed. A common mistake is to get out of the range of movement by bringing the upper arm too close to the body, or failing to "lead with the elbow." These types of throwing exercises can be

---

Warm-Up and Stretching

Arm circles—Squat with hands on hips—Sit-ups—Trunk rotations

		Distance	% Max.	Time
Aerobic Conditioning Run:	*Minimum*	0.5 mi.	75%	3–5 mins. (approx.)
	Goal	2.0 mi.	75%	15–16 mins. (approx.)

Strength Training (Universal Gym)—*Train Explosively!*

Circuit: 60 second station, rotate through circuit two times

Station #1—Bench Press, 6–10 reps
    2—Pull-ups, max 15 reps and Sit-ups
    3—Military Press, 6–10 reps
    4—Back Hyperextension, 10–15 reps
    5—Chin-ups on Y bar, 15 reps max
    6—Upright rowing, 10–15 reps

7—Lat Pulls, 10–15 reps
    8—Leg Press, 10 reps
    Toe Raises, 30 reps
    9—Bar Dips, 15 reps max
    10—Leg Extension, 10–15 reps
    11—Neck Extension, 10–15 reps
    12—Grip Exercise series

Stretching Exercises

FIGURE 9.1 *Off-Season Circuit for Junior High Football*

Warm-Up and Stretching

		Distance	% Max.	Time
Aerobic Conditioning Run: *Minimum*		0.5 mi.	75%	4–5 min. (approx.)
	Goal	2.0 mi	75%	15–16 min. (approx.)

Strength Training—Train Explosively!

Monday

Bench Press
10-10-8-6-4-2-2-2
(Start with more reps if you're
not already lifting. Heavy max.
reps are not necessary. Do
only once a week if at all.)

Squats
10-10-8-6-4-2-2-2
(Unnecessary to go down to
parallel.)

Toe Raises
8 sets, 30 reps

Tricep Extension
8-5-5-5-5

Curls
5 sets, 10 reps

Sit-Ups
5 sets, 10–20 reps

Neck Extension
4–6 sets, 10 reps

Bent Arm Pullover
5 sets, 10 reps

Shoulder Shrugs
5 sets, 10 reps

Stretching Exercises

Wednesday

Military Press
10-10-8-8-6-6-4-4

High Pulls or Cleans (Similar
to Upright Rows)
5-4-3-3-3-2
(Great for interior linemen.)

Tricep Extension
8-5-5-5-5

Curls
5 sets, 10 reps

Sit-Ups
5 sets, 10–20 reps

Neck Extension
4–6 sets, 10 reps

Bent Arm Pullover
5 sets, 10 reps

Inclines or Dips
(Could be substituted for
Military Press)

Shoulder Shrugs
5 sets, 6 reps

Friday

Bench Press
10-10-8-8-5-5-5-5
(Start with more reps if
you're not already lifting.
Heavy max. reps are not
necessary. Do only once a
week if at all.)

Squats
10-10-8-8-5-5-5-5
(Unnecessary to do down
to parallel.)

Toe Raises
8 sets, 30 reps

Tricep Extension
8-5-5-5-5

Curls
5 sets, 10 reps

Sit-Ups
5 sets, 10–20 reps

Bent Arm Pullover
5 sets, 10 reps

Shoulder Shrugs
5 sets, 8 reps

FIGURE 9.2 *Off-Season Conditioning Program for Junior High Football*

Warm-Up and Stretching

		Distance	% Max.	Time
Aerobic Conditioning Run: *Minimum*		1.0 mi.	75%	7–8 min. (approx.)
	Goal	2.0 mi.	75%	14–15 min. (approx.)

Strength Training—Train Explosively!

Monday

Bench Press
10-10-8-8-6-6-4-4

Half-Squat
8-8-6-6-4-4-3-3

Wednesday

Incline
10-10-8-8-6-6

High Pulls or Cleans
5-4-3-3-3-2

Friday

Bench Press
10-10-8-5-3-3-3-3

Half-Squat
8-8-8-6-6-4-4-4

FIGURE 9.3 *Off-Season Conditioning Program for Offensive and Defensive Backs* (H.S.–College)

(Continued)

Monday	*Wednesday*	*Friday*
Toe Raises 8 sets, 30 reps	Speed Exercise 6 sets, 10–15 reps	Toe Raises 8 sets, 30 reps
Speed Exercise (30 lbs. max.) 6 sets, 10–15 reps	Sit-Ups 5 sets, 14 reps	Speed Exercise 6 sets, 10–15 reps
Sit-Ups 5 sets, 10 reps	Grip Exercises 305 sets	Sit-Ups 5 sets, 18 reps
Neck Extension 4–6 sets, 10 reps		Neck Extension 4–6 sets, 10 reps
Grip Exercises 3–5 sets		Grip Exercises 3–5 sets

Optional

Split Squats, Jumping Squats, Wrist Curls, Good Mornings, Tricep Extensions, Shoulder Shrugs

Stretching Exercises

FIGURE 9.3 *(Continued)*

Warm-Up and Stretching

		Distance	% Max.	Time
Aerobic Conditioning	Run: *Minimum*	0.5 mi.	75%	4–5 mins. (approx.)
	Goal	2.0 mi.	75%	15–16 mins. (approx.)

Strength Training—Train Explosively!

Monday	*Wednesday*	*Friday*
Bench Press 8-8-6-3-2-1-1-4-4	Incline Press 10-10-8-8-6-6	Bench Press 10-10-8-8-5-5-5-5
Half-Squat 8-8-6-3-2-1-1-4-4	Dips 10-10-8-8-6-6 (Military Press can be substituted for Dips and trained as Incline Press.)	Half-Squat 10-10-8-8-5-5-5-5
Toe Raises 8 sets, 30 reps		Toe Raises 8 sets, 30 reps
Tricep Extension 8-5-5-5-5	High Pulls or Cleans 8-6-5-5-5	Tricep Extension 8-5-5-5-5
Sit-Ups 5 sets, 10 reps	Tricep Extension 8-5-5-5-5	Sit-Ups 5 sets, 18 reps
Neck Extension 4–6 sets, 10 reps	Sit-Ups 5 sets, 14 reps	Neck Extension 4–6 sets, 10 reps
Grip Exercises 3–5 sets	Grip Exercises 3–5 sets	Grip Exercises 3–5 sets

Optional

Lat Pulls, Upright Rowing, Presses Behind Neck, Leg Presses, Wrist Curls, Good Mornings, Curls, Shoulder Shrugs
Linebackers and Defensive Ends—Frontal Delts, Wrist Curls

Stretching Exercises

FIGURE 9.4 *Off-Season Conditioning Program for Linemen and Linebackers* (H.S.–College)

Warm-Up and Stretching

	Distance	% Max.	Time
Aerobic Conditioning Run: *Minimum*	1.0 mi.	75%	7–8 min. (approx.)
Goal	2.0 mi.	75%	14–15 min. (approx.)

Strength Training—Train Explosively!

Monday and Friday

Bench Press
10-10-8-8-6-6-4-4

Half-Squat
8-8-6-6-4-4-3-3

Throwing Pullover
5 sets, 10 reps

Toe Raises
8 sets, 30 reps

Sit-Ups, Twisting
5 sets, 10 reps
(18 on Friday)

Throwing Motion (wall pulley)
5 sets, 10 reps

Wrist Roller or Wrist Curl
5 sets

Neck Extension
5 sets, 10–15 reps

Wednesday

Dips
6 sets, 10 reps

Incline Press
8-8-8-6-6-6-4-4

High Pulls or Cleans
8-6-5-5-5

Toe Raises
8 sets, 30 reps

Sit-Ups, Twisting
5 sets, 14 reps

Throwing Motion (wall pulley)
5 sets, 10 reps

Wrist Roller or Wrist Curl
5 sets

Neck Extension
5 sets, 10–15 reps

Optional
Upright Rowing, Bent Over Rowing, Lat Pull, Curls, Tricep Extension, Incline Press.

Throwing

Stretching

FIGURE 9.5 *Off-Season Conditioning Program for Quarterbacks* (H.S.–College)

Warm-Up and Stretching

Strength Training—Train Explosively!

Monday and Friday

Half Squat
6 sets, 8 reps

Leg Extension (from flexed position)
5–6 sets, 10 to 15 reps

Toe Raises
8 sets, 30 reps

Wall Pulley (kicking motion)
5 sets, 10 to 15 reps

Sit-Ups
5 sets, 10 reps (18 on Friday)

Wednesday

Leg Extension
5 sets, 10 to 15 reps

High Pulls or Cleans
8-6-5-5-5

Toe Raises
8 sets, 30 reps

Wall Pulley (kicking motion)
5 sets, 10 to 15 reps

Sit-Ups
5 sets, 14 reps

FIGURE 9.6 *Off-Season Conditioning Program for Kickers* (H.S.–College)

(Continued)

Monday and Friday	*Wednesday*
Leg Lifts 5 sets, 10 reps	Leg Lifts 5 sets, 10 reps
Bench Press 5 sets, 8 reps	Military Press 5 sets, 8 reps

Optional
Lat Pull, Bench Press, Incline Press, Bent Over Rowing

Kicking

		Distance	*% Max.*	*Rest*	*Reps*
Anaerobic Exercise	Run:	100 yds.	100%	30 secs.	5-10

Stretching Exercises

FIGURE 9.6 *(Continued)*

Warm-Up and Stretching

Aerobic Conditioning (3/Week)	*Distance*	*% Max.*
Run:	1.5–2.0 mi.	75%

Strength Training—Training Explosively!

Monday		*Thursday*	
Bench 8–10 sets 10-10-8-8-6-6-6-6-4-4	*Upright Rowing* 5 sets, 10 reps	*Military Press* 8–10 sets 10-10-8-8-6-6-6-6	*Leg Press* or *Rack Squat* 6–10 sets
Squat 8–10 sets 8-8-8-8-6-6-6-6	*Sit-Ups* 5 sets, 10 reps	*Bar Dips* 8–10 sets 10-10-8-8-8-8	*Sit-Ups* 5 sets, 14 reps
Toe Raises 8–10 sets, 30 reps	*Specialty Exercise*	*Tricep Extension* 8-5-5-5-5	*Specialty Exercise*
Tricep Extension 8-5-5-5-5		*Friday*	
Tuesday		*Press Behind Neck* 8–10 sets	*Toe Raises* 8–10 sets
Incline 8–10 sets 10-10-8-8-6-6-4-4	*Good Morning* 5 sets, 8 reps	*High Pulls* or *Cleans* 5 sets 8-6-5-5-5	*Bent Over Row* 5 sets, 10 reps
High Pulls or *Cleans* 5–6 sets 8-6-5-5-5	*Sit-Ups* 5 sets, 12 reps	*Deadlift* 5-4-3-2-1	*Sit-Ups* 5 sets, 16 reps
Toe Raises 8–10 sets, 30 reps	*Neck Extension* 5 sets, 10–15 reps	*Good Morning* 5 sets, 10 reps	*Neck Extension* 5 sets, 10–15 reps

FIGURE 9.7 *High-Intensity Off-Season Conditioning Programs for College Football Player "A"*

(Continued)

Saturday

Bench 8–10 sets 10-10-8-6-4-2-1-1-4-4	*Toe Raises* 8–10 sets, 30 reps
Dumbbell Bench 5 sets 8-8-8-6-6	*Tricep Extension* 8-5-5-5-5
Squat 8–10 sets 8-8-8-6-4-2-1-1-4-4	*Sit-Ups* 5 sets, 16 reps
Specialty Exercise	
Stretching Exercises	

FIGURE 9.7 *(Continued)*

Warm-Up and Stretching

Aerobic Conditioning (3/Week)	*Distance*	*% Max.*
Run:	1.5–2.0 mi.	75%

Strength Training—Train Explosively!

Monday

Behind Neck Press 10 sets 10-10-10-8-8-6-6-4-4-2	(S)	*Sit-Ups* 5 sets, 12 reps	
Dips 10-10-8-8-8-6-6-6-6	(D)	*High Pulls* or *Cleans* 8-6-5-5-5	
Bent Over Rowing 5 sets, 10 reps		*Neck Extension* 5 sets, 10–15 reps	

Tuesday

Bench 12-12-10-10-6-6-4-4-2-2	(D)	*Curls* 5 sets, 14 reps	
Squat 8-8-8-8-6-6-4-4-2-2		*Sit-Ups* 5 sets, 14 reps	
Calves 10 sets, 30 reps		*Tricep Extension* 8-5-5-5-5	

Thursday

Dips 10-10-8-8-6-6-6-6-4-4	(S)	*Sit-Ups* 5 sets, 16 reps	
Incline 10-10-10-10-8-8-6-6-6-6	(D)	*Specialty Exercise*	
Curls 5 sets		*Neck Extension* 5 sets, 10–15 reps	

FIGURE 9.8 *High-Intensity Off-Season Conditioning Programs for College Football Player "B"*

(Continued)

Friday

Military Press   (D)   *Curls*
10-10-8-8-6-6-4-4-4-4-2-2   5 sets, 10 reps

Squat   *Sit-Ups*
8-8-8-8-6-6-4-4-4-4-2-2   5 sets, 18 reps

Calves   *Tricep Exension*
10 sets, 30 reps

Stretching Exercises

FIGURE 9.8 *(Continued)*

trained with the regular weight training program, 10-15 repetitions, 5-6 sets.

The advantages of using such a circuit are efficient use of time, total body development in terms of increased strength, and cardiovascular as well as muscular endurance. This type of program can be completed in approximately 60 minutes, three times per week. It is advisable for the coach to conduct an instructional session with young athletes concerning proper techniques and goals for weight training. The circuit system can be varied from three to 25 or 30 stations. When a large number of stations are used, exercises for agility or quickness may also be included.

For the more highly competitive programs, strength training programs are offered with consecutive sets of each exercise. Fewer reps (1–8) will be used with the noncircuit programs. Special programs that can be used in the off-season are also included. Such programs include training regimens of more than the traditional every-other-day approach. For brief periods (4–8 weeks) some athletes will be able to condition for five or more days per week. The authors identify this as "high-intensity" training and certainly *do not recommend* such a regimen for most athletes.

A series of off-season conditioning programs follows. They are appropriate for junior high, high school, or college-level conditioning. The collegiate programs could indeed be used by professionals. Some of the programs are specified according to position.

PRE-SEASON

As the pre-season approaches there will be a dramatic shift in the conditioning approach. The shift will be from aerobic to anaerobic conditioning and from slow-speed, heavy-resistance strength conditioning to fast-speed, high-repetition strength training.

The major objectives of pre-season conditioning are the development of *anaerobic power*, *explosive strength*, and *injury prevention*. For those athletes who have been on an off-season program, the shift is to more intensive anaerobic training and high-speed strength training. The resistance must be reduced to produce the latter objective. Agility drills and quick reaction training increase.

For athletes who have not engaged in an off-season program, rapid strength and anaerobic development can be hastened by the use of a special circuit. High-repetition, high-speed strength training should be emphasized. Anaerobic training can be very unpleasant and fatiguing for the athlete who has not developed good aerobic power to aid recovery from sprints. The authors recommend a *test* at the beginning of the pre-season period to determine if the athlete can meet the aerobic GOAL listed in the off-season programs (2.0 mi. in 14–16 mins.). This will quickly determine which players have not followed the aerobic portion of the off-season conditioning program.

Specificity of conditioning becomes the major consideration as the football player approaches the playing season. If some kind of "training camp" is held pre-season, coaches and athletes may desire to shift to a pre-season regimen before going to the training camp.

A variety of pre-season programs are offered from junior high through college level.

Warm-Up and Stretching

Strength Training—Train Explosively!

Monday–Friday	*Wednesday*
Bench Press	*Military Press*
10,10,8,8,8,8	10,10,8,8,8,8
Squats	*High Pulls* or *Cleans*
8,8,8,8,8,8	8,5,5,4,3
Toe Raises	*Curls*
8 sets, 30 reps	5 sets, 10 reps
Tricep Extension	*Tricep Extension*
5 sets 8,5,5,5,5	5 sets 8,5,5,5,5
Sit-Ups	*Sit-Ups*
5 sets, 10–20 reps	5 sets, 10–20 reps
Neck Extension	*Neck Extension*
4–6 sets, 10 reps	4–6 sets, 10 reps

Anaerobic Conditioning

	Distance	% Max.	Rest	Reps	Times/Week
Run:	100 yds.	100%	30 secs.	5–10	3–5

Stretching Exercises

FIGURE 9.9 *Preseason Conditioning Program for Junior High Football*

Warm-Up and Stretching

Strength Training—Train Explosively!

Monday	*Wednesday*	*Friday*
Bench Press	*Incline*	*Bench Press*
2 weeks	2–4 weeks	2 weeks
10-10-10-10-8-8	10-10-8-8-8-8	10-10-10-10-10-10-8-8
Half-Squats	(Alternate, Single set	*Half-Squats*
2 weeks 6 sets, 8 reps	and Double Sit-ups	2–4 weeks 6 sets, 8 reps
Toe Raises	*High Pulls* or *Cleans*	*Toe Raises*
8 sets, 30 reps	8-6-5-5-5	8 sets, 30 reps
Speed Exercise (30 lbs. max.)	*Speed Exercise*	*Speed Exercise*
6 sets, 10–15 reps	6 sets, 10–15 reps	6 sets, 10–15 reps
Sit-Ups	*Sit-Ups*	*Sit-Ups*
5 sets, 10 reps	5 sets, 14 reps	5 sets, 18 reps
Neck Extension	*Grip Exercise*	*Neck Extension*
4–6 sets, 10 reps	3–5 sets	4–6 sets, 10 reps
Grip Exercise		*Grip Exercise*
3–5 sets		3–5 sets

Optional
Split Squats, Jumping Squats, Wrist Curls, Good Mornings

FIGURE 9.10 *Preseason Conditioning Program for Offensive and Defensive Backs* (H.S.–College)

(Continued)

Anaerobic Conditioning (daily)

	Distance	% Max.	Rest	Reps
Run	100 yds.	100%	30 secs.	10–15

Stretching Exercises

FIGURE 9.10 *(Continued)*

Warm-Up and Stretching

Strength Training—Train Explosively!

Monday	Wednesday	Friday
Bench Press	Incline Press	Bench Press
10-10-8-8-8-8	2 weeks 10-10-8-8-8-8	2 weeks 10-10-8-8-8-8
Half-Squat	Dips	Half-Squat
10-10-8-8-8-8	2 weeks 10-10-8-8-8-8	10-10-8-8-8-8
Toe Raises	(Military Press can be	Toe Raises
8 sets, 30 reps	substituted for Dips and	8 sets, 30 reps
	trained as Incline Press.)	
Tricep Extension	High Pulls or Cleans	Tricep Extension
8-5-5-5-5	8-6-5-5-5-5	8-5-5-5-5
Sit-Ups	Tricep Extension	Sit-Ups
5 sets, 10 reps	8-6-5-5-5	5 sets, 18 reps
Neck Extension	Sit-Ups	Neck Extension
4–6 sets, 10 reps	5 sets, 14 reps	4–6 sets, 10 reps
Grip Exercise	Grip Exercise	Grip Exercise
3–5 sets	3–5 sets	3–5 sets

Optional
Lat Pulls, Upright Rowing, Presses Behind Neck, Leg Presses, Wrist Curls, Good Mornings, Curls

Linebackers and Defensive Ends—Frontal Delts, Wrist Curls

Anaerobic Conditioning (daily)

	Distance	% Max.	Rest	Reps
Run:	100 yds.	100%	30 secs.	10

Stretching Exercises

FIGURE 9.11 *Preseason Conditioning Program for Linemen and Linebackers* (H.S.–College)

Warm-Up and Stretching

Strength Training—Train Explosively!

Monday & Friday	*Wednesday*
Bench Press 2 weeks 10-10-10-10-8-8	*Dips* 6 sets, 10 reps
Half-Squat 2–4 weeks 8-8-8-8-8-8	*Incline Press* 8-6-5-5-5
Throwing Pullover 5 sets, 10 reps	*High Pulls* or *Cleans* 8-6-5-5-5
Toe Raises 8 sets, 30 reps	*Toe Raises* 8 sets, 30 reps
Sit-Ups, Twisting 5 sets, 10 reps (18 on Friday)	*Sit-Ups, Twisting* 5 sets, 14 reps
Throwing Motion (wall pulley) 5 sets, 10 reps	*Throwing Motion* (wall pulley) 5 sets, 10 reps
Wrist Roller or *Wrist Curl* 5 sets	*Wrist Roller* or *Wrist Curl* 5 sets
Neck Extension 5 sets, 10 to 15 reps	*Neck Extension* 5 sets, 10 to 15 reps

Optional
Upright Rowing, Bent Over Rowing, Lat Pull, Curls, Triceps Extension, Incline Press

Anaerobic Conditioning (daily)

	Distance	*% Max.*	*Rest*	*Reps*
Run:	100 yds.	100%	30 secs.	10–15

Throwing

Stretching Exercises

FIGURE 9.12 *Preseason Conditioning Program for Quarterbacks* (H.S.–College)

Warm-Up and Stretching

Strength Training—Train Explosively!

Monday & Friday	*Wednesday*
Half-Squat 6 sets, 8 reps	*Leg Extension* 5 sets, 10 to 15 reps
Leg Extension (from flexed position) 5–6 sets, 10 to 15 reps	*High Pulls* or *Cleans* 8-6-5-5-5
Toe Raises 8 sets, 30 reps	*Toe Raises* 8 sets, 30 reps
Kicking Motion (wall pulley) 5 sets, 10 to 15 reps	*Kicking Motion* (wall pulley) 5 sets, 10 to 15 reps
Sit-Ups 5 sets, 10 reps (18 on Friday)	*Sit-Ups* 5 sets, 14 reps

FIGURE 9.13 *Preseason Conditioning Program for Kickers* (H.S.–College)

(Continued)

Monday & Friday	Wednesday
Leg Lifts	*Leg Lifts*
5 sets, 10 reps	5 sets, 10 reps
Bench Press	*Military Press*
5 sets, 8 reps	5 sets, 8 reps

Optional
Lat Pull, Bench Press, Incline Press, Bent Over Rowing

Running, Kicking: Stretching should follow each weight training session.

Anaerobic Conditioning (daily)

	Distance	% Max.	Rest	Reps
Run:	100 yds.	100%	30 secs.	10–15

Kicking

Stretching Exercises

FIGURE 9.13 *(Continued)*

IN-SEASON

As detailed in Chapter 8, aerobic condition and strength can be maintained with a minimum time expenditure during the in-season period. Anaerobic conditioning should be continued *daily*, either at the conclusion of practice or within practice. During the brief and intense pre-season period aerobic conditioning has been minimized.

The major objectives of in-season conditioning are the continuation of *anaerobic* conditioning (daily), maintenance of *aerobic power* and

Warm-Up and Stretching

Aerobic Conditioning

	Distance	% Max.	Times/Week
Run:	1.0–1.5 mi.	75%	2

Strength Training (2 per week) — *Train Explosively!*

Leg Press, Leg Extension, or Half-Squat	3 sets,	10 reps
Bench, Military Press, or Incline	3 sets,	10 reps
Neck Extension	3 sets,	10 reps
High Pulls or Upright Rowing	3 sets,	5–8 reps
Throwing Exercise (quarterbacks)	3 sets,	10 reps

Stretching Exercises

Note:

Anaerobic Conditioning (daily)

	Distance	% Max.	Rest	Reps
Run:	50 yds.	100%	30 secs.	10–20

FIGURE 9.14 *In-Season Circuit for Junior High Football*

Warm-Up and Stretching

Aerobic Conditioning

	Distance	% Max.	Times/Week
Run:	1.5 mi	75%	2

Strength Training (1–2 per week)—Train Explosively!

Backs and Receivers

Choice of Jumping Squat,
High-Speed Machine, Half-Squat
3 sets, 10 reps

Speed Exercise
3–5 sets, 10 reps

Incline or *Bench Press*
3–5 sets, 8 to 10 reps

Leg Extension
3 sets, 10 reps

Upright Rowing or *High Pull*
3 sets, 5 to 10 reps

Wrist Roller or *Wrist Curl*
3–5 sets

Neck Extension
3 sets, 10 to 15 reps

Interior Linemen and Linebackers

Choice of Jumping Squat,
High-Speed Machine, Half-Squat
3–5 sets, 8 to 10 reps

Incline, Bench, or *Military Press*
3–5 sets, 8 to 10 reps

Lat Pull
3 sets, 10 reps

Leg Extension
3 sets, 10 reps

High Pulls or *Cleans*
8-6-5

Upright Rowing
3 sets, 10 reps

Neck Extension
3 sets, 10 to 15 reps

Defensive Linemen may wish to replace Upright Rowing with Forearm Shiver exericse.

Center can add Snaps with a weighted football, and/or centering motion with a wall pulley, Mini Gym, etc.

Quarterbacks

Leg Extension or *Half-Squat*
3 sets, 10 reps

Throwing Motion (wall pulley)
3 sets, 10 reps

Wrist Roller
3 sets (both directions)

Incline or *Bench Press*
3 sets, 8 to 10 reps

Jumping Squats
3 sets, 12 reps

Kickers

Leg Extension
3 sets, 10 to 15 reps
(from flexed position, if possible)

Kicking Motion (wall pulley)
3–5 sets, 10 reps

Toe Raises
3–5 sets, 30 reps

Leg Curl
3 sets, 10 to 20 reps

Anaerobic Conditioning (daily)

	Distance	% Max.	Rest	Reps
Run:	50 yds.	100%	30 secs.	10–20

Stretching Exercises

FIGURE 9.15 *In-Season Conditioning Programs for Football* (H.S.–College) *strength*, and *prevention* of injuries. Aerobic and strength conditioning can be reduced to two sessions weekly. Strength training will emphasize fast-speed, high-repetition work as was used in the preseason period. The specialty exercises can be added if not already used. The reader is referred to Chapter 6 for preventive exercises designed to reduce injury.

The coach should look for ways to condition the team within the regular practice session. The two-minute drill, for example, is an excellent overload for the anaerobic system. Many agility or other football drills can serve the purpose of developing skills and conditiong at the same time. There are many ways to save that ever-precious time that must be spent on skills development and strategy and still condition a football team.

A variety of brief in-season conditioning programs are offered from junior high to college level.

SPECIALTY EXERCISES AND PROGRAMS

Specialty exercises for football can serve two purposes: 1) they may be designed to strengthen the muscles involved in a specific football skill, or 2) they may be designed to aid in the rehabilitation of injury. An example of the latter is diagonal movements of the legs done with pulleys following knee surgery. Such action is designed to strengthen the lateral movements of players after surgery or injury.

Among the football specialty exercises that have been used in programs in this chapter are:

Kicking Motion (with wall pulley)

The kicking motion is produced with the pulley attached to the ankle. An upright support is recommended so that the kicker can hold himself in the upright position during the exercise.

Throwing Motion

The throwing motion is done with a football or a handle attached to the high wall pulley. Quarterbacks training with this exercise should be certain that the stance and throwing motion are imitated exactly. The wrist turns *out* when releasing a football, and this motion should be emphasized.

Bent Arm Deltoid Raises

This exercise is done with a dumbbell, and the range of motion should imitate the "forearm rip." The exercise is used by linemen and running backs.

Defensive Tackles and Middle Guards

Power Clean and Press
8-5-5-5-5

Lying Tricep Extension
3 sets, 10 reps

Bench Press
3 sets, 8–12 reps

Upright Row
3 sets, 8–12 reps

Bent Over Row
3 sets, 8–12 reps

Wrist Roller
3 sets

Flankers and Split Ends

Speed Exercise
5 sets, 10 reps

Wrist Roller
5 sets

Neck Extension
5 sets, 10 reps

Bench Press
5 sets 8-8-6-6-6

Offensive Linemen

Power Clean
Reps 5-5-3-3-1

Squat
Reps 8-6-6-4-4

Dead Lift
Reps 5-5-3-3-1

Neck Extension
5 sets, 10 reps

FIGURE 9.16 *Strength Programs (Off-Season or Preseason) for Special Positions*

PHOTO 9.1   *Kicking Motion*

PHOTO 9.2 *Throwing Motion*

PHOTO 9.3 *Bent Arm Deltoid Raises*

Centering Motion

The movement is done with a pulley at ground level or as close to ground level as possible. The exercise is designed to aid in developing power for the longer snaps at center, and for speed in making the short snap. The motion desired should be imitated as exactly as possible. For the long snap, the arms are extended and greater resistance can be used. The short snap should be practiced at higher speed and less resistance.

State II (AN–LA) during the "two-minute offense" periods at the end of the first half and the game. Stage III (AER) comes into play primarily during the recovery phase or rest interval between plays.

Strength, explosive power, speed, agility, and flexibility are all important in good performance. In this chapter the authors have offered programs to develop all of the essential factors in football. The programs are designed for three levels (junior high school, high school, and college) during the off-season, pre-season, and in-season.

SUMMARY

Football is a predominately anaerobic game. The action involves State I (ATP–CP) almost entirely. Occasionally the demands of the game require

REFERENCES

1. Fracas, G. "Football." In *The Scientific Aspects of Sports Training*, ed. A. W. Taylor. Springfield, IL: Charles C. Thomas, (1975), pp. 137–162.

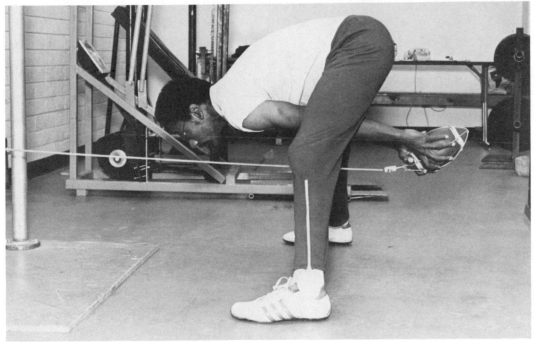

PHOTO 9.4 *Centering Motion*

2. Paige, Roderick R. *What Research Tells the Coach about Football*. Washington, D.C.: AAHPERD, 1973.

3. Riley, Daniel P. *Strength Training for Football: The Penn State Way*. West Point, NY: Leisure Press, 1978.

4. Stone, William J., and Kroll, William A. Unpublished research data, Arizona State University, 1977.

5. Ward, Bob et al. "Optimizing Human Performance Through Computerization of the Conditioning Program Design." *NSCA Journal* 4 (1982): 6–7, 9, 4].

10 Soccer

This chapter includes aerobic and anaerobic conditioning programs and strength building programs for soccer. In order to make the most effective use of the programs offered here, the reader is referred to Chapter 3 for the basis of aerobic and anaerobic training programs, Chapter 4 for the basis of strength programs, and Chapter 5 for the details of stretching programs. It is also recommended that the reader refer to Chapter 8 for the most efficient means of incorporating those objectives into a single workout. The programs are offered for off-season, pre-season, and in-season. The reader is also referred to the sample recording charts in the Appendix. These charts facilitate the measurement of the athlete's progress in the training program, and will also indicate the athlete's standing in regard to training goals.

Soccer is clearly the most popular sport in the world. It has also elicited more emotion from spectators than any other game. Deaths associated with soccer games are not uncommon, and in 1969 a full-scale war erupted over a playoff series between Honduras and El Salvador. The Salvadoran army invaded Honduras and over 2,000 lives were lost. Since the publication of the first edition of this book, soccer has grown tremendously in popularity in this country. This is especially true of youth sports leagues, which in turn has led to the development of high school teams and leagues. The North American Soccer League (NASL) and the Major Indoor Soccer League (MISL) also reflect the growing interest in soccer at the professional level. There is every indication that soccer will continue to grow in popularity as a spectator sport and in number of participants in the future. Soccer is also one of the most thoroughly researched sports in terms of energy demands of the activity, physiological characteristics of players, and training routines.[5]

One of the most obvious characteristics of soccer is that it is very aerobic in nature. In international rules the game is played in two 45-minute halves of nearly continuous play. Ninety minutes of action was not sufficient to determine a winner in the 1978 World Cup final between Argentina and Holland. A 30-minute overtime was played resulting in a total of 120 minutes of continuous action, halted only by the half time and a rest period after the regulation time had expired. Extensive studies indicate that nearly 90 percent of the movement is aerobic and that forwards, who range over the most territory, will cover five to nine miles per game.[5] The aerobic power of soccer players is very high among team sports athletes, averaging from 56-66 ml/kg/min. for VO_2 max (maximal oxygen uptake).

Explosive power and speed are also important factors in soccer performance. About 10 percent of the time in the game the soccer player is involved in anaerobic bursts which include: sprinting over short distances, jumping explosively, and making movements that require much agility and flexibility.[5] Strength development in the legs is obviously important because of the requirements for jumping, turning, kicking, and quick starts. A strong neck and upper body should also be developed, not only to improve the performance of some soccer skills (heading), but also to prevent injuries.

Soccer is certainly one of the most physically demanding of team sports with players averaging heart rates of 155-165 during play. This converts to approximately 75 percent of maximal aerobic power for the more active positions. Although highly skilled players can reduce the energy expenditure by accurate passing and good position play, soccer obviously is a game that requires a significant conditioning effort in addition to the skills and strategies that must be developed. Conditioning efforts should be directed toward developing aerobic power, agility and flexibility, anerobic power (sprinting), and strength.

YOUTH SPORTS LEAGUES

Most soccer participants in the United States are concentrated in youth sports leagues. Because of the late arrival of soccer as a popular sport, most of the current players are in the six to sixteen year-old range. The greatest concentration of youth sports performers is usually in the seven to twelve year-old bracket. The programs offered in this chapter are not designed or intended to be used by very young athletes. Most youth sports leagues are philosophically committed to fun, widespread participation, and low-key competition.

Intense training is usually not recommended for most athletes prior to the junior high school level.

Youth sports performers in soccer can benefit, however, from low-key conditioning programs, which are usually dominated by running activities. Aerobic power can and should be developed in young soccer players by "warm-up" runs, continuous practice sessions, and lead-up games which also include a great deal of aerobic movement. Sprint races and relays can become a fun part of practice to aid in the development of speed and anaerobic power. Calisthenics and flexibility exercises can precede practice or game so that the young athlete begins to learn the importance of a good warm-up and stretching routine. Such efforts are restricted to the pre-season and in-season periods. They should not become a burden for the

---

Warm-Up and Stretching

		Distance	% Max.	Time (approx.)
Aerobic Conditioning　　Run: *Goal*		3–5 mi.	75%	21:00–35:00

Strength Training—Train Explosively!

Monday & Friday	*Wednesday*
Bench Press 10, 10, 8, 8, 6, 6, 4, 4	Military Press 10, 10, 8, 8, 6, 6, 6, 6
Half Squat 8, 8, 8, 6, 6, 6, 4, 4	Leg Press 8, 8, 8, 6, 6, 6, 4, 4
Leg Extension 10, 10, 8, 8, 8, 8	Leg Extension 10, 10, 8, 8, 8, 8
Leg Curl 5 Sets, 10 Reps	Leg Curl 5 Sets, 10 Reps
Leg Lifts 5 Sets, 10–15 Reps	Leg Lifts 5 Sets, 10–15 Reps
Sit-Ups 5 Sets, 10–15 Reps	Sit-Ups 5 Sets, 10–15 Reps
Toe Raises 6 Sets, 30 Reps	Toe Raises 6 Sets, 30 Reps
Throw-In Motion 5 Sets, 10 Reps	Throw-In Motion 5 Sets, 10 Reps
Kicking Motion 5 Sets, 10 Reps	Kicking Motion 5 Sets, 10 Reps
Upright Rowing 5 Sets, 10 Reps	Upright Rowing 5 Sets, 10 Reps
High Knee Lift 5 Sets, 10 Reps	High Knee Lift 5 Sets, 10 Reps

Stretching Exercises

FIGURE 10.1 *Off-Season Conditioning Program for Soccer*

youthful competitor and the coach needs to keep in mind that the goals of youth sports are fun, participation, and low-key competition.

OFF-SEASON

The off-season conditioning program should concentrate on developing aerobic power and strength. Both of these capacities require significant amounts of time for training, which should be available during the off-season. Off-season conditioning should consist of running for aerobic development. Strength training will be aimed primarily at developing leg power and upper body power, particularly arm, shoulder, and neck strength. Greater resistance and fewer repetitions will be characteristic of the strength training in the off-season. Figure 10.1 offers an off-season conditioning program for soccer. Flexibility training continues year round.

PRE-SEASON

The object of the pre-season program is to bring the soccer player to peak playing condition in as brief a time as possible. Training becomes more intense during the pre-season period. There is a shift to more intense aerobic intervals and to anaerobic conditioning. The shift in strength training is toward higher speed, greater repetition, low-resistance training. A pre-season conditioning program for soccer is offered in Figure 10.2.

IN-SEASON

The objectives of the in-season conditioning program are to maintain strength and aerobic conditioning, continue anaerobic conditioning, and prevent injuries. Strength and aerobic conditioning sessions are reduced to one or two per week, while anaerobic conditioning is maintained daily.

Warm-Up and Stretching

Aerobic Conditioning (3/Week)

	Distance	% Max.	Rest	Reps
Run:	2.0 mi.	75%	—	—
or	0.5 mi.	90%	3 mins.	3–5

Strength Training—Train Explosively 3 Days per Week

Bench Press or Military Press
3–6 sets, 8–15 reps

Half Squat, Jumping Squat or Leaper
3–6 sets, 8–15 reps

Leg Extension
6 sets, 10–15 reps

Leg Curl
5 scts, 10–15 reps

Leg Lifts
5 sets, 10–15 reps

Sit-Ups
5 sets, 10–25 reps

Upright Rowing
5 sets, 10 reps

Throw-In Motion
5 sets, 10 reps

Kicking Motion
5 sets, 10 reps

High Knee Lift
5 sets, 10 reps

Toe Raises
6 sets, 30 reps

Anaerobic Conditioning

	Distance	% Max.	Rest	Reps	Times/Week
Run:	50–100 yds.	100%	30–60 secs.	5–10	2–3

Stretching Exercises

FIGURE 10.2 *Pre-Season Conditioning Program for Soccer*

Warm-Up and Stretching

Aerobic Conditioning (2/Week)

		Distance	% Max.	Rest	Reps
Run:		2–3 mi.	75%	—	—
or		0.5 mi.	90%	3 mins.	3

Strength Training—Train Explosively 1 or 2 days per week

Bench Press or Military Press 2–5 sets, 8–15 reps	Sit-Ups and/or Leg Lifts 2–5 sets, 10–15 reps
Half Squat, Jumping Squat or Leaper 2–5 sets, 8–15 reps	Throw-In Motion and/or Kicking Motion 2–5 sets, 10–15 reps
Leg Extension 2–5 sets, 8–15 reps	High Knee Lift 5 sets, 10–15 reps
Leg Curls 2–5 sets, 8–15 reps	

Anaerobic Conditioning

	Distance	% Max.	Rest	Reps	Times/Week
Run:	75 yds.	100%	45 secs.	5–10	4–5

Stretching Exercises

FIGURE 10.3 *In-Season Conditioning Program for Soccer*

A relatively short expenditure of time is sufficient to maintain strength and aerobic conditioning.

The coach should be alert for opportunities to condition within the regular practice session. Aerobic conditioning can be maintained or improved with continuous play such as scrimmages with no time-outs. Various high-speed passing and/or ball handling drills, as well as supplemental sprints, can be used to develop anaerobic conditioning.

An in-season conditioning program for soccer is offered in Figure 10.3.

SUMMARY

Approximately ninety percent of the game of soccer is played aerobically. Despite that fact, the game also calls for occasional bursts of speed and high levels of agility. Leg strength and power are very important for the soccer player.

In this chapter the authors have developed off-season, pre-season, and in-season conditioning programs. The programs are aimed at the development of the major factors contributing to soccer performance.

REFERENCES

1. Beim, George. *Principles of Modern Soccer.* Boston: Houghton Mifflin Co., 1977.
2. Clues, Andrew, and Jack, David. *Soccer for Players and Coaches.* Englewood Cliffs, N.J.: Prentice-Hall, 1980.
3. Fardy, Paul S. "Scientific Basis of Training for Soccer." In Edmund J. Burke, ed., *Toward an Understanding of Human Performance.* 2d ed. Ithaca, N.Y.: Mouvement Publications, 1980.
4. Micheli, Lyle, and Leard, John. "Conditioning for Soccer." *Coach & Athlete* 43 (May/June, 1981): 32–36.
5. Reilly, Thomas. *What Research Tells the Coach about Soccer.* Washington, D.C.: AAHPERD, 1979.

11

Basketball

In this chapter the authors include aerobic and anaerobic conditioning programs and strength-building programs for basketball. In order to make the most effective use of the programs offered here, the reader is referred to Chapter 3 for the basis of aerobic and anaerobic training programs, to Chapter 4 for the basis of strength programs, to Chapter 5 for the basis of warm-up and stretching programs, and to Chapter 8 for the most efficient means of incorporating those objectives into a single workout. The training is offered as off-season, pre-season, and in-season programs at three levels. The three levels include junior high school, senior high school, and college training programs. The reader is also referred to the sample recording charts shown in the Appendix. These charts will facilitate the measurement of the athlete's progress on the training program and will also indicate the athlete's standing in regard to training goals.

Unlike football, basketball involves all three energy stages (I-III) during the active portion of the game. Basketball can be a very *aerobic* game although it also includes many *anaerobic power* (Stage I) skills in jumping, shooting, and rebounding. The continuous nature of the game and the constant movement required of high-caliber play contribute toward making basketball a game of high endurance. Occasional bursts of fast-break basketball rely on *anaerobic* capacity and this, too, must be considered in the conditioning program. No other sport described in this book, with the possible exception of hockey, requires as many energy capacities *during play* as does basketball. The athlete or coach must be prepared to condition for the specific requirements of the game.

The level and style of play can greatly influence the pace of the game and thus the energy expenditure. Obviously a "run-and-gun," fast-break offense involves higher levels of both aerobic and anaerobic power. The slow-paced, deliberate style of play places less demand on physical conditioning, but it is still necessary.

The authors have found that the 24-second clock in the NBA generally ensures that the action will be fast paced, but "breaks" in the action will be more frequent. Timing studies indicate that the ball tends to stay in play an average of 30 seconds before the clock stops for an out-of-bounds or foul.[3] Closer examination of the data, however, indicated that play or action did not stop when the clock was off for five seconds or less.[4] Players would continue down court on a turnover or go into the transition with a non-shooting foul. As a result, it was determined that the ball remained in play an average of 65 seconds before there was as long as a ten-second rest interval. In high school and college basketball the ball can generally remain in play longer before a shot will be made, thus decreasing the chance of a break in action for a free throw or out-of-bounds.

Strength training is an important part of basketball conditioning because of the need for leg strength and power for jumping and rebounding. Movements on the floor must be quick, explosive, and agile. Upper body and grip strength are necessary in rebounding. Increased leg power may add inches to the player's jump, and greater strength will aid in controlling the ball—neither of these, of course, can replace proper positioning, timing, or shooting skill. Many young basketball players are in need of greater strength and power to go with their natural height. It has been found that teams that discontinue weight training during the season lose vertical jumping ability,[5] also that a variety of strengthening regimens will increase vertical jumping power, including jumping practice alone.

Strength training for basketball players carries one note of caution from the authors: *Very tall players (6'8" and above) should be careful to keep*

175

the back straight when doing Squats. Because of the long upper body, it is possible to get the bar too far from the base of support (feet) by leaning forward, thus putting undue pressure on the lower back. The Squat should not be omitted from basketball programs, however, because of its value in building leg strength and power.

Improving the aerobic capacity of basketball players will mean that they can play longer and more vigorously. Teams that rely on a "running" game should benefit greatly from increased aerobic capacity. Studies with the Phoenix Suns of the NBA indicate that a year-round program of aerobic training can pay dividends not only in higher aerobic capacity, but also in improved performance. The Suns as a team consistently test higher in aerobic capacity than the results reported for many other NBA teams. Since the inception of the "running" program at the conclusion of the 1977 season, they have appeared in the playoffs every year to date. By training for anaerobic power, the basketball player should also be better able tolerate all-out effort.

capacity and strength. Both of these capacities require time for conditioning and that time is available during the off-season. The aerobic conditioning should proceed until the athlete meets the listed GOAL. The young athlete with expectations of a college or professional basketball career should learn to condition year round.

Strength training for basketball should always be explosive but the off-season exercises are done with greater resistance which slows the movement slightly. For most exercises, maximum repetitions will be done in the range of 1-10 RM, usually on the upper end of that range for greater muscular endurance. Strength exercises that are done primarily for muscular endurance (Good Mornings or Toe Raises) are done with low resistance and high repetition during the off-season.

The authors recommend that off-season programs be done in circuit training style. This enables conditioning for all aspects of basketball to be included in a single training session. It also concentrates the conditioning and reduces the amount of time spent in each session.

OFF-SEASON

During the off-season period a great deal more time can be spent in conditioning for both aerobic

PRE-SEASON

During the preseason period there is a shift to more intense (anaerobic) conditioning and strength training more specific to the nature of basketball.

Warm-Up and Stretching

		Distance	% Max.	Time (approx.)
Aerobic Conditioning	Run: *Minimum*	1.0 mi.	75%	7– 8:00 mins.
	Goal	2.5 mi.	75%↑	18–20:00 mins.

Strength Training (2 per Week)—Train Explosively!

Squat 6–8 sets, 10 reps	Toe Raises 8–10 sets, 30 reps	Ankle Exercise 3–5 sets
Bench Press 6–8 sets, 10 reps	Wrist Roller and/or Wrist Curls 3–5 sets	Pulldown Close Grip 3–5 sets
*Good Morning or Stiff-legged Dead Lift 3–5 sets, 10 reps	Cleans 5 sets, 8-5-5-3-3	Military Press 3–6 sets, 10 reps
Jumping Squats 4–5 sets, 10–15 reps	Throwing Pullover 3–5 sets, 10 reps	

Stretching Exercises

*Use a very light weight for this exercise (approx. 50% of 10–15 RM).

FIGURE 11.1 *Off-Season Conditioning Program for Junior High Basketball*

Warm-Up and Stretching

		Distance	% Max.	Time (approx.)
Aerobic Conditioning	Run: *Minimum*	1.0 mi.	75%	6:30– 7:00 mins.
	Goal	3.0 mi.	75%↑	20:00–24:00 mins.

Strength Training—Train Explosively!

Monday & Friday

Squats   Jumping Squats (or Fast Speed Machine)
8 sets (A) 10-10-8-8-6-6-6-6   5 sets, 10–15 reps
       (B) 10-10-8-8-6-6-4-4

Bench Press   *Good Morning (or Stiff-legged Dead Lift)
8 sets 10-10-8-8-6-6-4-4   5 sets, 10 reps
       10-10-8-6-4-2-6-6
       (Last 6's done explosively with   *Shooting Exercise
       moderately heavy weight)   5 sets, 10–15 reps

Bent Over Rowing (with dumbbells)   Lat Pull Down
5 sets 10-10-8-8-8   5 sets, 8–10 reps

Grip	Toe Raises	Stretching & Ankle
3–5 sets	8 sets, 30 reps	Exercises
		3–5 sets, 10 reps

Wednesday

Rack Squat	Shooting Exercise	Toe Raises
3–5 sets, 8-8-5	5 sets, 10–15 reps	8 sets, 30 reps
Cleans	Lat Pull Down	Stretching & Ankle
5 sets, 8-5-5-3-3	5 sets, 8–10 reps	Exercises
		3–5 sets, 10 reps
Incline Press	Grip	
6–8 sets, 8-8-6-6-6-6	3–5 sets	
Split Squats, Jumping	Leg Extension	
5 sets, 6 reps each leg	3 sets, 6–12 reps	

Stretching Exercises

     *Use a very light weight for this exercise (approx. 50% of 10–15 RM).

FIGURE 11.2 *Off-Season Conditioning Program for High School and College*

Both the speed of contraction and the number of repetitions should be increased for the strength training. The objective is to increase the local muscular endurance by high-speed, high-repetition training.

     The anaerobic conditioning at this point in the season will be more intense than during the in-season period. The objective is to train the anaerobic (Lactic Acid) system, and this is the most rigorous of all training techniques. This kind of training prepares the player to tolerate high level bursts (fast breaks) in a continuous sequence.

     Pre-season conditioning should be designed to bring the basketball player to playing condition in the shortest possible time. The player should be expected to meet the goals set down in Figures 11.2 and 11.3 for aerobic power. The more intense conditioning occurs just prior to the season so that the player will be at top condition for the first time just as the season opens. This is designed to reduce the potential for fatigue or staleness in the latter part of the season. The coach who is particularly pressed for time can use the circuit training technique both pre-season and in-season.

     Pre-season programs are offered at the junior high, high school, and college levels.

Warm-Up and Stretching

Strength Training—Train Explosively!

Bench Press
3–5 sets, 10–15 reps

Ankle Exercise
3–5 sets

*Jumping Squat
3–5 sets, 10–20 reps

Pulldown Close Grip
3–5 sets, 10–15 reps

Wrist Roller and/or Wrist Curl
3–5 sets

Military Press
3–5 sets, 10–15 reps

*Throwing Pullover
3–5 sets, 10 reps

*Good Morning or Stiff-legged Dead Lift
3–5 sets, 10–20 reps

		Distance	% Max.	Rest	Reps
Anaerobic Conditioning	Run: *Minimum*	220 yds.	90%↑	2 mins.	5
	Maximum	440 yds.	90%↑	3 mins.	5

		Time	Rest	Reps
or: (Anaerobic Conditioning—*Indoor*)				
	Run: Continuous sprints	30 secs.	2 mins.	5
	(floor length)	45 secs.	3 mins.	5

Stretching Exercises

*Use very light weight for this exercise (approx. 50% of 10–15 RM).

FIGURE 11.3 *Pre-Season Conditioning Program for Junior High Basketball*

Warm-Up and Stretching

Strength Training—Train Explosively!

Monday & Friday

Bench Press
6 sets, 10 reps

Toe Raises
8 sets, 30 reps

Shooting Exercise
5 sets, 10–15 reps

Jumping Squats
5 sets, 10–15 reps

High Pull
5 sets, 8-6-5-5-5 reps

Lateral Raises (with dumbbells)
5 sets, 15 reps

Wrist Roller
8 sets

Throwing Pullover
5 sets, 10 reps

Ankle Exercise
3–5 sets

Wednesday

Bent Over Rowing
6 sets, 10 reps

Wrist Curl
6 sets, 30 reps

Pulldown Close Grip
6 sets, 8-6-6-6-6 reps

Split Squats
6 sets, 10–15 reps

Upright Rows
5 sets, 8-6-5-5-5 reps

Shooting Exercise
5 sets, 10–15 reps

Toe Raises
8 sets, 30 reps

Military Press
6 sets, 10 reps

Ankle Exercise
3–5 sets

		Distance	& Max.	Rest	Reps
Anaerobic Conditioning	Run: *Minimum*	220 yds.	90%↑	2 mins.	5–10
	Maximum	440 yds.	90%↑	3 mins.	5–10

FIGURE 11.4 *Pre-season Conditioning Program for High School and College Basketball*

(Continued)

		Time	Rest	Reps
or: (Anaerobic Conditiong—*Indoor*)				
	Run: Continuous sprints	30 secs.	2 mins.	5–10
	(floor length)	60 secs.	3 mins.	5–10

Stretching Exercises

   *Light weight and fast explosive repetitions should be used for all resistance exercises.

FIGURE 11.4 *(Continued)*

IN-SEASON

The purpose of in-season conditioning for basketball is to maintain a high level of aerobic and anaerobic condition, and strength and muscular endurance. With the exception of anaerobic conditioning, two sessions per week will maintain aerobic capacity and strength. Anaerobic conditioning should be continued *daily* during the season either during or after practice.

The strength training program is abbreviated by use of only two or three sets of each exercise at high repetition. High-speed training is emphasized, as it is more specific to the explosive nature of basketball skills (jumping, rebounding, and quick movements). Injury prevention is the major reason for ankle exercises in the strength program during the in-season period.

Basketball offers many opportunities for conditioning during the in-season period and within the regular practice. Continuous scrimmage with no time-outs is an excellent way of maintaining aerobic power. Repeated fast break drills or other high-speed drills such as passing or dribbling can be used for anaerobic conditioning. Rebound drills can develop leg power as well as rebounding skills if they are done in continuous fashion. One-on-one or two-on-one drills are also good conditioners as well as skill drills if the players are involved in continuous play. Most coaches employ a wide

---

Warm-Up and Stretching

		Distance	% Max.
Aerobic Conditioning	Run:	1.5 mi.	75%

**Strength Training—Train Explosively!*

Jumping Squats (with light weights) 2–3 sets, 12 reps	Shooting Exercise 2–3 sets, 10–12 reps
Grip Exercise 3–5 sets	Ankle Exercise 3–5 sets

Optional Exercises
Military Press, Lateral Raises with dumbbells, Lat Pulls, Bent Over Rowing, Bench Press

		Time	Rest	Reps
Anaerobic Conditioning (Daily)				
	Run: Continuous sprints	20–30 secs.	1 min.	5–8
	(floor length)			

Stretching Exercises

   *Light weight and fast explosive repetitions should be used for all resistance exercises.

FIGURE 11.5 *In-Season Conditioning Program for Junior High School Basketball*

Warm-Up and Stretching

		Distance	*% Max.*
Aerobic Conditioning	Run:	2.0 mi.	75%

*Strength Training—Train Explosively!

Jumping Squats (or Fast Speed Machine)
2–3 sets, 10–15 reps

Wrist Curls
3 sets

Shooting Exercise
2–3 sets, 10–12 reps

Ankle Exercise
2–3 sets

Lat Pulldowns
2–3 sets, 10–12 reps

Optional Exercises

Military Press, Lateral Raises with dumbbells, Bent Over Rowing, Bench Press, Split Squats.

Anaerobic Conditioning (Daily)	*Time*	*Rest*	*Reps*
Run: Continuous sprints (floor length)	20–30 secs.	1 min.	5–10

Stretching Exercises

  *Light weight and fast explosive repetitions should be used for all resistance exercises.

FIGURE 11.6 *In-Season Conditioning Program for High School and College Basketball*

PHOTO 11.1 *Shooting Exercise*

range of skill drills that can double as conditioning exercises by making them continuous or high-speed.

SPECIALTY EXERCISES

Shooting Exercise

The exercise is done with a ten-pound dumbbell (smaller athletes may use a five-pound dumbbell).

The exercise begins with the dumbbell held at the forehead and the elbow pointed straight ahead. The exact range of motion for shooting the basketball is followed, turning over or flexing the wrist at the end of the movement.

Dorsiflexion of the Foot

(See Chapter 5.)

Jumping Squats

These may be done using a light barbell or dumbbells. The weight is usually held at the shoulders in front of the body, but may be held behind the head. The athlete then takes the normal position for jumping and leaps vertically with a maximum effort. This may be done with the legs split slightly (or one foot in front of the other).

PHOTO 11.2 *Jumping Squats*

PHOTO 11.2   *Jumping Squats (Dumbell)*

SUMMARY

Basketball is generally an aerobic game that is punctuated with short bursts (Stage I, ATP–CP) of action and occasionally intense Stage II involvement (AN–LA). It is one of the more demanding sports since it involves all three of the energy mechanisms during play. In addition, it also requires explosive power, strength, flexibility, and agility at high levels.

In this chapter the authors have offered programs to develop all of the essential factors in basketball. The programs are designed for off-season, pre-season, and in-season at three levels (junior high school, high school, and college).

REFERENCES

1. Anderson, Bob. "Stretching for Basketball." *NSCA Journal* 2 (1980): 22–25.
2. Hoolahan, Paul. "Strength and Conditioning for Basketball: The University of North Carolina Program." *NSCA Journal* 2 (1980): 20–21.
3. Kroll, William A. "Conditioning for Basketball." *NSCA Journal* 4 (1983): 24–26.
4. Stone, William J. Unpublished research data, Arizona State University, 1978.
5. Yarr, A. D. "Basketball." In *The Scientific Aspects of Sports Training*, A. W. Taylor, ed. Springfield, IL: Charles C. Thomas 1975, pp. 199–221.

12

Hockey

This chapter contains year-round conditioning programs for hockey. The programs are designed for the off-season, pre-season, and in-season periods. In order to make the most effective use of these programs the reader is referred to Chapter 3 for the basis of aerobic and anaerobic training programs, to Chapter 4 for the basis of strength programs, to Chapter 5 for the basis of warm-up and stretching exercises, and to Chapter 8 for the most efficient means of incorporating those objectives into a single workout. The reader is also referred to the sample recording charts offered in the Appendix. These charts will facilitate the measurement of progress of the athlete in the training program, and will indicate the athlete's standing in regard to the training goal.

In the opening chapter of this book, ice hockey was used to illustrate the importance that superior conditioning can mean in a team game. The example, the reader may recall, involved the USSR versus "Team Canada" is a series begun during the 1970s. Although the Soviets had been successful against U.S. collegiate teams in the past, no one seriously expected the Soviet national team to be a difficult opponent for the NHL All-Star group making up Team Canada. The pattern of the games was set early in the series with the Canadians dominating play early, the Soviets shifting the momentum in the second period, and then typically out-skating the NHL players in the third period.

The superior conditioning of the USSR team was no accident. Koloskov, a Russian sports scientist, has outlined the premise behind the Soviet hockey conditioning[3]. He maintains that the most important trend in modern international hockey is an increase in the number of plays which puts a premium on: speed, endurance, strength, and agility. If a team can generate more plays and more shots on goal, and the goalie's stop percentage remains constant, the team will score more goals!

Hockey is one of the most vigorous of team sports and requires a great deal of physical conditioning. Like basketball, it requires a high level of *aerobic* and *anaerobic* conditioning. Like basketball, it also contains a great deal of continuous activity (aerobic) interrupted by anaerobic bursts of speed. Approximately two-thirds of the maximal aerobic capacity is the average expenditure of energy for the hockey player, who skates an average of 2.5 miles per game.[5] At least 20 to 25 percent of the game is played in the *anaerobic* mode, which makes the game so intense.[2] One of the reasons for the Soviet success against the NHL players is that they had conditioned their team to go anaerobically for 65 to 75 percent of the time. Average heart rates range from 87 to 92 percent of max during game action.

Strength training is also a significant factor in the preparation for hockey. Leg power is necessary for quick acceleration, while upper body strength and arm and wrist strength are important in controlling the puck, shooting, and checking opponents.

There are two unique aspects to hockey from a training standpoint. Since lines can be changed on the fly, action can be more continuous and at a higher aerobic level than in many other sports. Fatigued players do not have to wait for time-out to be relieved, thus a high level of aerobic play can be maintained almost constantly. Players may remain on the ice in the range of one to four minutes, depending upon position. The forward line does more high-speed skating and covers more distance, while the defense men can pace their energy expenditure and remain on the ice longer.

Another unique aspect of hockey is the movement on ice. This raises the question of specificity in training. In most sports, movement on the court or on the field is by foot, thus running is an excellent and specific training mode. The inevitable question is, should hockey players condition aerobically and anaerobically on ice? The answer obviously is yes, if it is available. If ice is not available to the hockey player in the off-season, running is a good substitute training mode. Many hockey players may prefer to train aerobically by running during the off-season.

Since hockey requires a high aerobic and anaerobic power and a great deal of arm strength and leg power, the training regimen must be very rigorous, and year-round conditioning is almost essential to develop the kinds of capacities needed to play the game. Young athletes with career aspirations in hockey should become accustomed to year-round training by the time they reach the high school level.

OFF-SEASON

The off-season conditioning program should concentrate on developing aerobic power and strength. Both of these capacities require large amounts of time for training and that time should be available during the off-season. Off-season conditioning should consist of running (skating preferred) for

---

Warm-Up and Stretching

	Distrance	*% Max.*	*Time (approx.)*
Aerobic Conditioning Run: *Goal*	3 mi.	75%↑	20–24:000 mins.

Strength Training—Train Explosively!

Monday & Friday	*Wednesday*
Bench Press 6–10 sets 10-10-8-8-6-6-4-4-2-2	Incline or Military Press 6–8 sets 10-8-8-6-6-4-4
Half-Squat 6–10 sets 8-8-8-6-6-4-4-4-2-2	Bar Dips 6–8 sets 10-10-8-8-6-6
Toe Raises 6–8 sets, 30 reps	Toe Raises 6–8 sets, 30 reps
Good Morning or Stiff-legged Dead Lift 5 sets, 10 reps	Good Morning or Stiff-legged Dead Lift 5 sets, 10 reps
Upright Rowing 5 sets, 10 reps	Clean 5 sets 8-5-5-3-3
Slap Shot Motion 5 sets, 10 reps	Slap Shot Motion 5 sets, 10 reps
Back Hand or Reserve Slap Shot Motion 5 sets, 10 reps	Back Hand or Reverse Slap Shot Motion 5 sets, 10 reps
Sit-Ups (twisting) 5 sets, 10–20 reps	Sit-Ups (twisting) 5 sets, 10–20 reps
Ankle Exercise 3–5 sets	Ankle Exercise 3–5 sets
Wrist Roller and/or Wrist Curl 3–5 sets	Wrist Roller and/or Wrist Curl 3–5 sets
Neck Extension 3–5 sets, 10 reps	Neck Extension 3–5 sets, 10 reps

Optional Exercises

Bent Arm Pullover, Bent Over Rowing, Leg Extension, Tricep Extension, Lat Pull, Curl, Leg Curl, High Knee Lift, Leg Thrust.

Stretching Exercises

FIGURE 12.1 *Off-Season Conditioning Program for Hockey*

aerobic development. Strength training will be aimed primarily at developing leg power and upper body power, particularly arm, shoulder, and wrist strength. Greater resistance and fewer repetitions will be characteristic of the strength training in the off-season. Figure 12.1 offers an off-season conditioning program for hockey.

PRE-SEASON

The objective of the pre-season program is to bring the hockey player to peak playing condition in as brief a period of time as possible. Training becomes more intense during the pre-season period. There is a shift from aerobic to anaerobic conditioning, which must be done on the ice. The shift in strength training is toward higher speed, greater repetition, low-resistance training. A pre-season conditioning program for hockey is offered in Figure 12.2.

IN-SEASON

The objectives of the in-season conditioning program are to maintain strength and aerobic con-

dition, continue anaerobic conditioning, and prevent injuries. Strength and aerobic conditioning sessions are reduced to one or two per week, while anaerobic conditioning is maintained daily. A relatively short expenditure of time is sufficient to maintain strength and aerobic condition.

The coach should be alert for opportunities to condition within the regular practice session. High-speed stick handling or skating drills can be used repeatedly to develop anaerobic condition. Aerobic condition can be maintained or improved with continuous play such as scrimmages with no time-outs.

An in-season conditioning program for hockey is offered in Figure 12.3.

SUMMARY

Hockey is a high intensity game played in the upper one-third of the aerobic mode or fully anaerobic (Stages II and III). Like basketball, it requires all three energy mechanisms during play as well as explosive power and strength. A unique aspect of the game is the ability to change lines

---

Warm-Up and Stretching

Strength Training—Train Explosively!

Bench Press
3-6 sets, 8-15 reps

Half-Squat or Jumping Squat
3-6 sets, 8-15 reps

Toe Raises
3-6 sets, 30-75 reps

Good Morning or Stiff-legged Dead Lift
3-5 sets, 10 reps

Upright Rowing
3-5 sets, 10 reps

Slap Shot Motion
3-5 sets, 10 reps

Reverse Slap Shot Motion
3-5 sets, 10 reps

Sit-Ups (twisting)
3-5 sets, 10-50 reps

Ankle Exercise
3-5 sets, 10-20 reps

Wrist Roller and/or Wrist Curl
3-5 sets

Neck Extension
3-5 sets, 10 reps

Optional Exercises

Bent Arm Pullover, Bent Over Rowing, Leg Extension, Tricep Extension, Lat Pull, Curl, Leg Curl, High Knee Lift, Leg Thrust.

Anaerobic Conditioning		*Distance*	*% Max.*	*Rest*	*Reps*
	Skate:	Rink length	95%↑	15 secs.	8-12

Stretching Exercises

FIGURE 12.2 *Pre-Season Conditioning Program for Hockey*

Warm-Up and Stretching

Aerobic Conditioning (2 per week)	*Time*	*% Max.*	*Rest*	*Reps*
Skate:	10–15 mins.	75%↑	—	1

Strength Exercises—Train Explosively!

Bench Press 2–5 sets, 8–15 reps	Reverse Slap Shot Motion 2–3 sets, 10–15 reps
Upright Row 2–3 sets, 10 reps	Jumping Squat and/or Leg Extension 2–3 sets, 10–15 reps
Wrist Roller and/or Wrist Curl 2–3 sets	Ankle Exercise 2–3 sets
Slap Shot Motion 2–3 sets, 10–15 reps	

Optional Exercises

Bent Arm Pullover, Bent Over Rowing, Military Press, Incline Press, Bar Dips, Sit-ups, Toe Raises, Good Morning, Stiff-legged Dead Lift, Tricep Extension, Lat Pull.

Anaerobic Conditioning (Daily)	*Distance*	*% Max.*	*Rest*	*Reps*
Skate:	Rink length	100%	15 secs.	10–15

Stretching Exercises

FIGURE 12.3 *In-Season Conditioning Program for Hockey*

during play, thus keeping the intensity of the game high.

In this chapter the authors have offered programs to develop all of the essential conditioning factors in hockey. The programs are designed for off-season, pre-season, and in-season.

REFERENCES

1. Bjornarea, Bud. "Power Training for Hockey." *NSCA Journal* 3 (1981): 24–27.

2. Jette, Maurice. "The Physiological Basis of Conditioning for Ice Hockey Players." In *Toward an Understanding of Human Performance*, Edmund J. Burke, ed. 2d ed. Ithaca, NY: Mouvement Publications, 1980, pp. 68–71.

3. Kolosov, V. "Conditioning the Hockey Player." In *Ice Hockey: Research Developments and New Concepts*. Miami, FL: Symposia Specialists, Dec. 1978, pp. 31–35.

4. Landy, Fernand, and Orban, William A. R., eds. *Ice Hockey: Research Developments and New Concepts*. Miami, FL: Symposia Specialists, 1978.

5. Marcotte, Gaston, and Hermison, Ray, "Ice Hockey." In *The Scientific Aspects of Sports Training*, A. W. Taylor, ed. Springfield, IL: Charles C. Thomas, (1975).

13

Volleyball and Wrestling

This chapter contains year-round conditioning programs for volleyball and wrestling. The programs are designed for the off-season, pre-season, and in-season periods. The reader is referred to four previous chapters for the basis of the programs. Chapter 3 deals with aerobic and anaerobic conditioning, Chapter 4 with strength training, Chapter 5 with warm-up and stretching programs, and Chapter 8 with year-round conditioning. The latter chapter describes ways of most efficiently putting training objectives together into a single program. The reader is also referred to sample recording charts offered in the Appendix. These charts will facilitate the measurement of the athlete's progress on the training program and will indicate the athlete's standing in regard to training goals.

VOLLEYBALL

The movements required to play volleyball are very *anaerobic*. Setting, spiking, jumping, and blocking are all anaerobic power actions. The players are also in continuous movement throughout an entire game. This requires endurance of an *aerobic* nature and is particularly important in skilled play when a match may run into several hours. Conlee et al.[2] found that volleyball players had a slight predominance (56 percent) of fast twitch fibers (FT) but also had a reasonably high aerobic capacity (56ml/kg) compared to most team sports athletes. This means that the volleyball player is one who is capable of explosive leg power for the jump, and also able to maintain high-level play over several hours. The most active players must vertical jump an average of once every 43 seconds, sometimes jumping two or three

times successively. This requires a high level of *local muscular endurance* as well as a good aerobic training base. Volleys last an average of 8 to 10 seconds, with the ball staying in play a maximum of 20 seconds. There are approximately 10 to 12 seconds between serves. Depending upon the level of play, the contest may last an hour (junior high school) to two and one-half hours in high-level collegiate play.[1]

Strength training is extremely important in preparation for volleyball because of the explosive nature of the skills.[3] Power volleyball requires leg power for jumping, and arm and shoulder strength for spiking. The requirement for local muscular endurance in the legs is extreme. The repeated jumping that occurs in the game taxes not only the leg power of the player but also leg endurance.

The Japanese led the way with scientific studies of training, especially those designed to improve the vertical jump.[5] More recently, the Soviets and Cubans have emphasized endurance jumping and have also used depth jumping. Nearly a half century of research on vertical jump training suggests that there are many effective techniques to improve the vertical jumping ability of players in volleyball and basketball.[4] In addition to modern strength machines, free weights, rope skipping, depth jumping, and jump training have also proved to be effective.

Flexibility and agility are also very important for the volleyball player, since many of the "saves" come on dives or other out-of-position plays.

Highly skilled "power volleyball" can be deceptive to the casual observer. At first glance the game may not appear to be very physically demanding. Volleyball players and coaches, however, will quickly recognize the physical requirements described above. Year-round conditioning programs that meet those requirements are described in the next section.

Year-Round Conditioning

The objectives of the off-season program for volleyball are to develop the aerobic condition, and leg and arm power necessary to play the game properly. Considerably more time is available to the player to condition for those two objectives during the off-season than later in the year-round conditioning regimen. Considerable amounts of whole-body aerobic conditioning are combined with strength training for leg and arm power. There will be greater emphasis on the muscular endurance end of the strength-endurance continuum.

As the pre-season conditioning program develops the emphasis is on more intense aerobic conditioning. Aerobic intervals are recommended during this period in order to attain peak aerobic power at the beginning of the season. The major goal of pre-season conditioning should be to bring the athlete to top playing condition as rapidly as possible with a minimum expenditure of time. Strength training should continue to emphasize fast-speed, high-repetition work, with low resistance. The emphasis is on the development of local muscular endurance, particularly in the legs.

Since flexibility training has no seasonal emphasis, it will continue year round on a maintenance level.

Warm-Up and Stretching

	Distance	% Max.	Time (approx.)
Aerobic Conditioning Run:	1:5–3.0 mi.	75%	12:00–24:00 mins.

Strength Exercises—Train Explosively!

Monday & Friday	*Wednesday*
Bench 5–8 sets 10-10-8-8-6-6	Military or Incline Press 5–8 sets 10-10-8-8-6-6
Half-Squat 5–8 sets 8-8-8-8-6-6	Jumping Squat 5 sets, 8–15 reps
Toe Raises 5–8 sets, 30 reps	Toe Raises 5–8 sets, 30 reps
Throwing Pullover 5 sets, 10 reps	Throwing Pullover 5 sets, 10 reps
Wrist Curl 3–5 sets (25 front, 15 reverse)	Wrist Curl 3–5 sets (25 front, 15 reverse)
Serving Motion (with pulley) 3–5 sets, 10–15 reps	Serving Motion (with pulley) 3–5 sets, 10–15 reps
Spiking Motion (with pulley) 3–5 sets, 10–15 reps	Spiking Motion (with pulley) 3–5 sets, 10–15 reps
Reverse Curl 5 sets, 10 reps	Reverse Curl 5 sets, 10 reps
Sit-Ups and/or Leg Lifts 5 sets, 10–20 reps	Sit-Ups and/or Leg Lifts 5 sets, 10–20 reps
Set-shot Motion (with dumbbells) 5 sets, 10–15 reps	Set-shot Motion (with dumbbells) 5 sets, 10–15 reps

Optional Exercises
Tricep Extension, Leg Extension, Bent Over Rowing, Bent Arm Pullover, Ankle Exercise, Bar Dips.

Stretching Exercises

FIGURE 13.1 *Off-Season Conditioning Program for Volleyball*

During the in-season period, strength and aerobic condition can be maintained with a minimum expenditure of time. A two-day-a-week program will be sufficient to maintain strength and aerobic condition. Anaerobic conditioning for the legs must be continued daily during this period. During the in-season training program the coach can use skill drills or jumping drills as conditioners. Repeated spiking drills, for example, will serve not only for practicing the skill of spiking but also for developing leg power and endurance.

Year-round conditioning programs for volleyball are offered in Figures 13.1, 13.2 and 13.3.

SPECIALTY EXERCISES

Serving Motion (with wall pulley)

This motion in volleyball is identical to the Throwing Motion (with wall pulley) described in Chapter 4.

Spiking Motion (with wall pulley)

This movement is done with a slightly higher pulley than the serving motion so that the angular downward motion of the spike can be strengthened.

Warm-Up and Stretching

	Distance	% Max.	Rest	Reps
Aerobic Conditioning (Daily) Run:	880 yds.	85%↑	3 mins.	4–6

Strength Exercises—Train Explosively!

Monday & Friday	*Wednesday*
Bench Press 3–5 sets, 8–15 reps	Military or Incline Press 3–5 sets, 8–15 reps
Jumping Squats 3–5 sets, 10–15 reps	Jumping Squats 3–5 sets, 10–15 reps
Toe Raises 3–5 sets, 30–75 reps	Toe Raises 3–5 sets, 30–75 reps
Throwing Pullover 3–5 sets, 10–15 reps	Throwing Pullover 3–5 sets, 10–15 reps
Wrist Curls 3–5 sets (25 front, 15 reverse)	Wrist Curls 3–5 sets (25 front, 15 reverse)
Serving Motion (with pulley) 3–5 sets, 10–15 reps	Serving Motion (with pulley) 3–5 sets, 10–15 reps
Spiking Motion (with pulley) 3–5 sets, 10–15 reps	Spiking Motion (with pulley) 3–5 sets, 10–15 reps
Reverse Curl 3–5 sets, 10–15 reps	Reverse Curl 3–5 sets, 10–15 reps
Sit-Ups and/or Leg Lifts 3–5 sets, 10–50 reps	Sit-Ups and/or Leg Lifts 3–5 sets, 10–50 reps
Set-shot Motion (with dumbbells) 3–5 sets, 10–15 reps	Set-shot Motion (with dumbbells) 3–5 sets, 10–15 reps

Optional Exercises
Tricep Extension, Leg Extension, Bent Over Rowing, Bent Arm Pullover, Ankle Exercise, Bar Dips.

Stretching Exercises

FIGURE 13.2 *Pre-Season Conditioning Program for Volleyball*

Warm-Up and Stretching

Aerobic Conditioning (2 sessions/week)

	Distance	% Max.	Time (approx.)
Run:	2.0 mi.	75%↑	14–16:00 mins.

Strength Exercises—Train Explosively!

Monday & Wednesday

Bench Press
2–5 sets, 8–15 reps

Jumping Squat
2–3 sets, 10–20 reps

Serving Motion (with pulley)
2–3 sets, 10–15 reps

Spiking Motion (with pulley)
2–3 sets, 10–15 reps

Set-shot Motion (with dumbbells)
2–3 sets, 10–15 reps

Wrist Curls
2–3 sets, (25 front, 15 reverse)

Optional Exercises

Toe Raises, Throwing Pullover, Reverse Curl, Sit-Ups, Leg Lifts, Tricep Extension, Leg Extension, Bent Over Rowing, Bent Arm Pullover, Ankle Exercise, Military Press, Incline Press, Bar Dips.

Stretching Exercises

FIGURE 13.3 *In-Season Conditioning for Volleyball*

PHOTO 13.1 *Serving Motion*

Set Shot Motion (with dumbbells)

This is done by crouching in the normal SET position with dumbbells held in each hand. The athlete then extends the arms and body upward in the exact Set Shot motion.

SUMMARY

Volleyball involves many anaerobic power *movements using Stage I (ATP–CP). Since the movements are repeated, sometimes over a period of several hours,* aerobic *capacity is also highly important. Much attention is paid to* strength development in the legs and upper body. The volleyball player must also develop a high level of flexibility *and* agility *in order to keep the ball in play.*

The authors have offered off-season, preseason, and in-season conditioning programs for volleyball. Those programs are aimed at developing the major performance factors associated with volleyball.

PHOTO 13.2 *Set Shot Motion*

REFERENCES

1. Andresen, Rolf. "Consideration of a Volleyball Team." *Journal of the National Volleyball Coaches Association* 2 (1981): 19.
2. Conlee, Robert K. et al. "Physiological Effects on Power Volleyball." *The Physician and Sportsmedicine* 10 (1982): 93–97.
3. Disch, James G. "Theories of High Level Performance Applied to Volleyball: Performance Analysis and Conditioning." *Volleyball Technical Journal* 6 (1981): 69–74.
4. Lacy, Alan. "A Half-Century of Research on Vertical Jump Training." Unpublished research paper, Arizona State University, 1982.
5. Toyoda, H. *Training Theory for Volleyball in Japan.* Scarborough, Ont., Canada. Canadian Volleyball Association Publication, 1971.

WRESTLING

Wrestling is unique in at least two respects: 1) competition is divided into ten weight categories, and 2) the action is divided into specific intervals of time[8]. The former results in a major concern for selecting the ideal weight, and the latter in a range of wrestling time from three or five minutes at junior high school level to eight or nine minutes at the collegiate level. High school competition usually involves three two-minute intervals for a total wrestling time of six minutes. Since there is very little rest between wrestling intervals, a 3- to 9-minute period of action falls well within the *aerobic* Stage III energy mechanism. Numerous studies have confirmed the high aerobic capacity of wrestlers and the need to make endurance training a major portion of conditioning for wrestling.[9,10]

Wrestling is a sport that requires a great deal of both *aerobic* endurance and *strength*. Upper-body strength, agility, and rapid acceleration are specific needs of the wrestler. The total 9 minute block of time for a wrestling match must be considered an aerobic energy period, but within any one- to-three-minute sequence *anaerobic* output could be involved. The result is that the wrestler must be prepared for an aerobic work period with anaerobic bursts of activity coming at any time during the match. Year-round conditioning for wrestling should focus on those requirements of the sport. A year-round conditioning regimen is offered in the next section of this chapter.

Maintaining minimum body weight for classification is a major concern for the wrestler. Strength training must be done very selectively to avoid adding to body weight. The practice of dehydration, which is used by some wrestlers, is not recommended by the authors and is discussed in more detail in Chapter 7. Wrestlers as a group are very lean athletes. Research indicates that many of the most successful wrestlers are five percent body fat or less.[10] Since wrestlers spend so much time and effort reducing body weight to a minimum effective category, one should not attach a cause and effect to the success of very lean wrestlers. Among a group of very lean athletes (many begin the season at eight percent fat), successful wrestlers may be those who can tolerate body weight loss and continue to train and perform. Recent evidence supports the supposition that rapid weight loss and rehydration have a detrimental effect on muscle glycogen levels and strength.[7]

Year-Round Conditioning

During the off-season there should be concentration on the development of aerobic power and the development of strength in the upper body. More time can be expended on these two training objectives during the off-season when the time spent on skills development is reduced. The wrestler should be careful not to allow his body weight to increase significantly during the off-season. If it becomes necessary to combat weight problems, increased aerobic conditioning will help to control body weight. A combination of diet and exercise is the most effective means of reducing or maintaining body weight.

During the pre-season period aerobic training becomes more intense and strength training becomes increasingly geared to the development of muscular endurance. The major goal of the pre-season conditioning program is to bring the wrestler to peak physical condition in the briefest possible time. During this period the coach or athlete may desire to add specific anaerobic conditioning related to wrestling.

During the in-season period the major objective is to maintain high aerobic capacity with a minimum time expenditure. Strength training can be drastically reduced during the in-season period because strength is also developed by wrestling practice. There are many opportunities for the coach to include either aerobic or anaerobic conditioning in the wrestling practice session. Extending the duration of the practice wrestling bout produces an aerobic training effect. Short maximum bouts with brief rest intervals will increase the anaerobic training effect. Wrestlers are fortunate in that the activity itself produces a training effect for aerobic and anaerobic capacity as well as strength.

Year-round conditioning programs are offered for off-season, pre-season, and in-season in figures 13.4, 13.5, and 13.6. Flexibility training follows a year-round program that is consistently aimed at maintenance.

Warm-Up and Stretching

	Distance	% Max.	Time (approx.)
Aerobic Conditioning Run:	3–5 mi.	75%↑	21–40:00 mins.

Strength Training—Train Explosively!

Monday & Friday

Bench Press
8–10 sets 10-10-8-8-8-8-8-8

Half-Squat
8–10 sets 10-10-8-8-8-8-8-8

Toe Raises
8–10 sets, 30–50 reps

Wednesday

Incline Press
6–10 sets 10-10-8-8-8-8

Half-Squat
6–8 sets   10-10-8-8-8-8

Bar Dips
6–8 sets   10-10-8-8-8-8

FIGURE 13.4 *Off-Season Conditioning Program for Wrestling*

(Continued)

Good Morning, Stiff-legged Dead Lift,
or Hyperextension
5 sets, 10 reps

Curls
5 sets, 10–15 reps

Sit-Ups
5 sets, 10–50 reps

Bent Over Rowing
5 sets, 10–15 reps

Neck Extension
5 sets, 10 reps

Support Curl
5 sets, 10–15 reps

Wrist Roller and/or Wrist Curls
3–5 sets

Reverse Curl
5 sets, 10–15 reps

Toe Raises
8–10 sets, 30–50 reps

Good Morning, Stiff-legged Dead Lift,
or Hyperextension
5 sets, 10–15 reps

Curls
5 sets, 10–15 reps

Sit-Ups
5 sets, 10–50 reps

Bent Over Rowing
5 sets, 10–15 reps

Neck Extension
5 sets, 10 reps

Support Curl
5 sets, 10–15 reps

Wrist Roller and/or Wrist Curls
3–5 sets

Reverse Curl
5 sets, 10–15 reps

Optional Exercises

Military Press, Lat Pull, Bent Arm Pullover, Clean, Dead Lift, Tricep Extension, Leg Extension, Ankle Exercise.

Stretching Exercises

FIGURE 13.4 *(Continued)*

Warm-Up and Stretching

Aerobic Conditioning

	Distance	% Max.	Rest	Reps
Run:	880 yds.	95%↑	3 mins.	4–6

Strength Training—Train Explosively!

Monday-Wednesday-Friday

Bench Press or Dips
4–8 sets, 10-10-8-8-8-8

Half-Squat or Jumping Squat
4–8 sets, 10-10-8-8-8-8

Toe Raises
3–8 sets, 30–75 reps

Good Morning, Stiff-legged Dead Lift,
or Hyperextension
3–5 sets, 10–20 reps

Curls
3–5 sets, 10–25 reps

Sit-Ups
3–5 sets, 10–75 reps

Bent Over Rowing
3–5 sets, 10–20 reps

Neck Extension
3–5 sets, 10–20 reps

Support Curl
3–5 sets, 10–20 reps

Wrist Roller and/or Wrist Curl
3–5 sets

FIGURE 13.5 *Pre-Season Conditioning Program for Wrestling*

(Continued)

Monday-Wednesday-Friday

Reverse Curl
5 sets, 10–15 reps

Optional Exercises
Military Press, Lat Pull, Bent Arm Pullover, Clean, Dead Lift, Tricep Extension, Leg Extension, Ankle Exercise.

Stretching Exercises

FIGURE 13.5 *(Continued)*

Warm-Up and Stretching

Aerobic Conditioning

	Distance	% Max.	Time (approx.)
Run:	2–3 mi.	85%↑	14–22:00 mins.

Strength Training—Train Explosively!

Monday & Wednesday

Bench Press 2–5 sets, 10–25 reps	Curls and/or Reverse Curl 2–5 sets, 10–25 reps
Half-Squat 2–5 sets, 10–25 reps	Wrist Roller 2–5 sets
Bent Over Rowing 2–5 sets, 10–25 reps	Wrist Curls 2–5 sets, 25–40 reps

Optional Exercises
Military Press, Lat Pull, Bent Arm Pullover, Clean, Dead Lift, Tricep Extension, Leg Extension, Ankle Exercise.

Anaerobic Conditioning (daily)
(Specific anaerobic wrestling intervals should be selected by coach and athlete.), e.g.,

	Time	% Max.	Rest	Reps
Wrestle:	1 min.	100%	2 mins.	6–10
	3 mins.	95%	3 mins.	5–8

Stretching Exercises

FIGURE 13.6 *In-Season Conditioning Program for Wrestling*

SUMMARY

Wrestling is almost the perfect "interval" sport, with total wrestling time ranging between three and nine minutes. Wrestling is highly aerobic (Stage III) but is punctuated with anaerobic bursts of effort. Strength (whole body) is also important in wrestling, as are agility and speed.

The programs offered in this chapter are aimed at improving the major factors involved in wrestling. Programs are designed to be used in the off-season, pre-season, and in-season.

REFERENCES

6. Anderson, Bob. "Stretching for Wrestling." *NSCA Journal* 2 (1980): 18–22.

7. Houston, Michael E. et al. "The Effect of Rapid Weight Loss on Physiological Functions in Wrestlers." *The Physician and Sportsmedicine* 9 (1981): 73–78.

8. Leyshon, G. "Wrestling." In *The Scientific Aspects of Sports Training*, A. W. Taylor, ed. Springfield, IL: Charles C. Thomas, 1975, pp. 163–178.

9. Rasch, Phillip, and Kroll, Walter. *What Research Tells the Coach about Wrestling*. Washington, D.C.: AAHPER (1974).

10. Zambeaski, Edward J. "Wrestling and Research. In *Toward an Understanding of Human Performance*, Edmund J. Burke, ed. 2d ed. Ithaca, NY: Mouvement Publications, 1980.

14

Baseball and Softball

This chapter contains year-round conditioning programs for junior high, high school, and college baseball and softball. The programs are designed for the off-season, pre-season, and in-season periods. The reader is referred to three previous chapters for the basis of the programs. Chapter 3 deals with aerobic and anaerobic conditioning; Chapter 4 with strength training; Chapter 5 with warm-up, stretching, and flexibility; and Chapter 8 with year-round conditioning. The latter chapter also includes ways of most efficiently putting training objectives together in a single program.

Baseball and softball are very *anaerobic* games. With the exception of the pitcher and catcher, players engage in brief bursts of effort requiring primarily acceleration, power, and speed. On defense, the actions of the pitcher and catcher are more frequent but still anaerobic.

Most of the conditioning efforts and much of past research in baseball has focused on the pitcher.[5] In a series of recent studies on major leaguers, Coleman[1, 2] found pitchers to be taller, heavier, and fatter on the average than players at other positions. They also tended to have less upper body strength but greater leg strength than other players. Since the pitcher must deliver 100 to 150 pitches per game at a rate of about two per minute, it is evident why the pitcher also desires local muscular endurance in the legs. Pitchers engage in considerably more aerobic conditioning than players at other positions. *Aerobic* training for baseball and softball players serves primarily to assist in recovery from anaerobic performance and is more essential for pitchers and catchers. Coleman's studies also revealed that baseball players in the major leagues have aerobic capacities only slightly lower than those of volleyball players or soccer professionals.[2] It has also been found that baseball players as a group are very

flexible, but are just slightly below the average college male in fatness.

Arm *strength* and leg *power* are very important, so strength training is directed primarily at those two areas. Baseball and softball players can benefit a great deal from strength training.

In order to gain maximum performance benefit from strength training, the authors recommend several principles for baseball and softball players: 1) Strength exercises should be done as close as possible to performance, speed, and range of motion. This is particularly important during the pre-season and in-season periods. 2) Practice of the skill (throwing, batting, or running) is recommended after the strength-building exercise. Only one set of ten reps is sufficient. 3) Strength *must* be maintained *during* the season to be effective. Unpublished research by Kroll indicates that throwing power actually *decreases* during a season of baseball without supplementary strength training.[4] Kroll's study was conducted with junior college athletes and Coleman[3] has recently confirmed those results with major league players. Not only was the strength training group stronger at the conclusion of the season, but they also had reduced body fat and increased muscle tissue. There was no loss in the range of motion for the stronger players.

Many athletes and coaches are adamant in their attitude that in-season strength training is not feasible, but it can be accomplished with an expenditure of very little time. The programs that follow are designed for year-round conditioning.

OFF-SEASON

The off-season program in most sports is directed toward developing aerobic power and strength.

Baseball and softball players should also be concerned with strength and power development but less concerned with aerobic development. Aerobic conditioning should be practiced by pitchers and catchers, while players at other positions ought to concentrate on anaerobic conditioning.

Off-season strength training should utilize greater resistance and fewer reps than pre- or in-season training. Major muscle groups should receive the greatest concentration at this time as well as injury preventive exercises (see Chapter 6). Incline Flys, Arm Circles, and Lateral Raises are recommended to strengthen the shoulder joint, thus reducing the potential for soreness or injury as a result of throwing. Specialty exercises are provided within the programs (see Figures 14.1 and 14.2).

Warm-Up and Stretching

Strength Training—Train Explosively!

Bench Press
5–8 sets, 10-10-8-6-4-2-1

Half-Squat
5–8 sets, 10-8-6-4-2-1

Military Press
5–8 sets, 10-10-8-8-6-4

Lat Pulls
5 sets, 10 reps

Sit-Ups
5 sets, 10–25 reps

Throwing Pullover and/or Throwing Motion (wall pulley)
5 sets, 10 reps

Toe Raises
5 sets, 30 reps

Hitting Motion
5 sets, 8–10 reps

Wrist Roller and/or Wrist Curl
3–5 sets

Aerobic Conditioning (pitchers and catchers)

	Distance	% Max.	Time (approx.)
Run:	2.0 mi.	75%↑	15–17 mins.

Optional Exercises

Arm Circles, Lateral Raises, Incline Flys, Leg Extension, Neck Extension, Bar Dips, Pitcher's specialty exercises are also optional.

Stretching Exercises

FIGURE 14.1 *Off-Season Conditioning Program for Junior High Baseball and Softball*

Warm-Up and Stretching

Strength Training—Train Explosively!

Monday & Friday

Bench Press
Mon.: 6–10 sets, 10-10-8-8-6-6-6-6
Fri.: 6–10 sets, 10-10-8-6-3-3-3-3-3

Half-Squat
Mon.: 6–8 sets, 8-8-8-6-6-6-6-6
Fri.: 6–10 sets, 8-8-8-6-4-4-4-4

Toe Raises
6–8 sets, 30 reps

Wednesday

Military Press
6 sets, 10-10-8-8-6-6

Dips
10-10-8-8-6-6

Jumping Squat (with light weight)
6 sets, 10–12 reps

Toe Raises
6–8 sets, 30 reps

FIGURE 14.2 *Off-Season Conditioning Program for High School and College Baseball and Softball*

(Continued)

Monday & Friday	*Wednesday*

Throwing Motion (wall pulley)
   or Throwing Pullover
5 sets, 6–10 reps each

Wrist Roller
3–5 sets

Sit-Ups, Twisting
5 sets, 10–20 reps

Wrist Curls
Palms up   25 reps
Palms down   15 reps

3–5 sets,   40 reps

Incline Flys, Arm Circles, and/or Lateral Raises
3–5 sets, 10 reps (These exercises are highly
recommended for preventing arm and
shoulder soreness.)

Hitting Motion (with pulley or weighted bat)
3–5 sets, 10 reps

Throwing Motion (wall pulley)
   or Throwing Pullover
5 sets, 6–10 reps each

Wrist Roller
3–5 sets

Sit-Ups, Twisting
5 sets, 10–20 reps

Wrist Curls
Palms up   25 reps
Palms down   15 reps

3–5 sets,   40 reps

Incline Flys, Arm Circles, and/or Lateral Raises
3–5 sets, 10 reps

Hitting Motion (with pulley or weighted bat)
3–5 sets, 10 reps

Pitchers

Speed Exercise
5 sets, 8–15 reps

Hip and Leg Motion
5 sets, 10 reps

Hip Extension or Hyperextension
5 sets, 10 reps

Optional Exercises

Leg Extension, Incline Press, Bent Arm Pullover, Neck Extension, Upright Rowing.

Aerobic Conditioning (pitchers and catchers)

	Distance	*% Max.*	*Time (approx.)*
Run:	3.0 mi.	75%	20–24:00 mins.

Stretching Exercises

FIGURE 14.2 *(Continued)*

Flexibility programs for baseball and softball can be initiated in the off-season, and then followed year round on a maintenance regimen.

PRE-SEASON

The objective of the pre-season program is to bring the player to peak condition in the briefest possible time. Training thus becomes more intense than at any other period in the year-round plan. Strength exercises are done at high speed with slightly less resistance than previously. Specificity should be stressed, and specificity exercises should be performed as closely as possible to the skills they mimic.

Pre-season programs are offered at the junior high, high school, and college levels (see Figures 14.3 and 14.4).

Warm-Up and Stretching

Strength Training—Train Explosively!

Bench Press	Lat Pull	Toe Raises
2–3 sets, 10–15 reps	2–3 sets, 10 reps	2–3 sets, 30 reps
Jumping Squat	Sit-Ups	Hitting Motion
2–3 sets, 10–15 reps	2–3 sets, 10–20 reps	2–3 sets, 10–15 reps
Military Press or Incline Press	Throwing Pullover and/or	Wrist Roller and/or
2–3 sets, 8–12 reps	Throwing Motion (with wall pulley)	Wrist Curl
	2–3 sets, 10–15 reps	2–3 sets

Aerobic Conditioning (pitchers and catchers)

		Distance	% Max.	Time (approx.)	
Run:		1.5 mi.	75%↑	10–12 mins.	

Anaerobic Conditioning

		Distance	% Max.	Rest	Reps
Run:		100 yds.	100%	30 secs.	8–10

Stretching Exercises

FIGURE 14.3   *Pre-Season Conditioning Program for Junior High Baseball and Softball*

Warm-Up and Stretching

Strength Exercises—Train Explosively!

Bench Press	Sit-Ups (twisting)	Arm Circles
3–5 sets, 8–12 reps	3–5 sets, 10–25 reps	3–5 sets, 10–30 reps
Jumping Squat	Speed Exercise	Lateral Raises
3–5 sets, 8–12 sets	3–5 sets, 10–25 reps	3–5 sets, 10–20 reps
Toe Raises	Bar Dips	Hitting Motion
3–5 sets, 30 reps	3–5 sets, 10 reps	3–5 sets, 10 reps
Throwing Motion	Throwing Pullover	Military Press
(with wall pulley)	3–5 sets, 10 reps	3–5 sets, 8–12 reps
3–5 sets, 10–20 reps	Incline Flys	Leg Extension
Wrist Roller and/or Wrist Curls	3–5 sets, 10–15 reps	3–5 sets, 10 reps
3–5 sets		

Aerobic Conditioning (pitchers and catchers)

		Distance	% Max.	Time (approx.)	
Run:	2.0 mi.	75%	75%↑	14–16:00 mins.	

Anaerobic Conditioning

		Distance	% Max.	Rest	Reps
Run:		100 yds.	100%	30 secs.	10–12

Stretching Exercises

FIGURE 14.4   *Pre-Season Conditioning Program for High School and College Baseball and Softball*

IN-SEASON

The objectives of in-season conditioning are to maintain anaerobic power and strength, and to prevent injuries. A minimum amount of time will enable athletes to meet all those objectives. For example, two or three sets of exercises at high speed and less resistance will maintain strength. Training, as such, once or twice a week, will enable one to maintain strength for an entire season. Aerobic (for pitchers and catchers) and anaerobic conditioning must also be maintained in season (see Figures 14.5 and 14.6).

Warm-Up and Stretching

Strength Training—Train Explosively!

Bench Press
2–3 sets, 10 reps

Jumping Squat
2–3 sets, 10–15 reps

Wrist Roller and/or Wrist Curl
3–5 sets

Throwing Motion (with wall pulley)
2–3 sets, 10–15 reps

Hitting Motion (with pulley or weighted bat)
2–3 sets, 10–15 reps

Optional Exercises

Leg Extension, Military Press, Throwing Pullover, Bar Dips, Toe Raises, Sit-Ups, Speed Exercise.

Aerobic Conditioning (pitchers and catchers)

	Distance	*% Max.*	*Time (approx.)*	
Run:	1.5 mi.	75%↑	10–12 mins.	

Anaerobic Conditioning

	Distance	*% Max.*	*Rest*	*Reps*
Run:	50 yds.	100%	15 secs.	8–10

Stretching Exercises

FIGURE 14.5 *In-Season Conditioning Program for Junior High Baseball and Softball*

Warm-Up and Stretching

Strength Training—Train Explosively!

Bench Press
2–3 sets, 10–15 reps

Jumping Squat
2–3 sets, 12–20 reps

Throwing Motion (with wall pulley)
2–3 sets, 10–20 reps

Wrist Roller and/or Wrist Curl
3 sets

Hitting Motion
2–3 sets, 10 reps

Incline Flys, Arm Circles, and/or Lateral Raises
2–3 sets, 10–20 reps

Optional Exercises

Leg Extension, Military Press, Throwing Pullover, Bar Dips, Toe Raises, Sit-Ups, Speed Exercise.

Aerobic Conditioning (pitchers and catchers)

	Distance	*% Max.*	*Time (approx.)*
Run:	2.0 mi.	75%↑	14–16:00 mins.

FIGURE 14.6 *In-Season Conditioning Program for High School and College Baseball and Softball*

(Continued)

Anaerobic Conditioning

		Distance	% Max.	Rest	Reps
Run:		50 yds.	100%	15 secs.	10-15

Stretching Exercises

FIGURE 14.6 *(Continued)*

SPECIALTY EXERCISES

Arm Circles

These are done with the arms extended straight out to the sides, making small circles in alternating directions. They may be done with no weight or with a light 5 to 15 pound) dumbbell. This exercise will help prevent shoulder soreness and will aid throwing power. (See Chapter 6, p. 000.)

Lateral Raises

These are done in the standing position by elevating (abducting) the extended arms straight out to the sides and directly overhead. (See Chapter 6, pp. 000.)

Incline Flys

These are performed on an inclined bench with dumbbells. The dumbbells are held with the arms extended directly overhead. They are then lowered until the arms are parallel to the ground. Sometimes a slight bend in the elbows is necessary in the lowered position. (See Chapter 6, p. 000.)

Pitcher's Hip Motion

This exercise is done by attaching a wall pulley to the thigh just above the knee. The hip motion is then imitated exactly.

Throwing Motion

(See Chapter 4.)

SUMMARY

Both baseball and softball are highly anaerobic games involving a series of highly skilled movements performed primarily in Stage I (ATP–CP). Aerobic power serves primarily to aid recovery from the anaerobic effort. Pitchers require the highest aerobic capacity among players. Strength and explosive power are very important to the baseball player, as are agility and flexibility.

This chapter contains programs designed to improve the major factors contributing to baseball and softball. The programs are designed for off-season, pre-season, and in-season periods.

REFERENCES

1. Coleman, A. Eugene. "Skinfold Estimates of Body Fat in Major League Baseball Players." *The Physician and Sportsmedicine* 9 (1981): 77–82.
2. Coleman, A. Eugene. "Physiological Characteristics of Major League Baseball Players." *The Physician and Sportsmedicine* 10 (1982): 51–57.
3. Coleman, A. Eugene. "In-Season Strength Training in Major League Baseball Players." *The Physician and Sportsmedicine* 10 (1982): 125–126, 129–132.
4. Kroll, William A. "The Effects of an In-Season Weight Training Program on the Throwing Power of Junior College Baseball Players." Master's thesis, Arizona State University, 1974.
5. Reiff, Guy G. *What Research Tells the Coach about Baseball*. Washington, D.C.: AAHPERD, 1971.

PHOTO 14.1 *Pitcher's Hip Motion*

15

Swimming

This chapter contains year-round conditioning programs for swimming. The programs are designed for the off-season, pre-season, and in-season periods. The reader is referred to four previous chapters for the basis of the programs. Chapter 3 deals with aerobic and anaerobic conditioning, Chapter 4 with strength training, Chapter 5 with stretching, and Chapter 8 with year-round conditioning. The latter chapter also describes ways of most efficiently putting training objectives together into a single program. The reader is also referred to the sample recording charts offered in the Appendix. These charts will facilitate the measurement of the athlete's progress in the training program and will indicate the athlete's standing in regard to the training goal.

Swimming and track and field are unique compared to other team sports listed in Part II. The two areas represent the epitome of aerobic, anaerobic, and, in some cases, strength and power performances. Conditioning is a major aspect in preparation for both swimming and track and field. Entire books have been written on training and conditioning for both sports. The authors could not, within the limitations of a single chapter, expect to lay out a day-by-day, week-by-week conditioning program for swimming or track. They have, however, attempted to develop a basic and cohesive year-round conditioning program for both sports.

The authors have found swimming and track coaches to be the most scientific practitioners among coaching professionals. The United States has a long history of excellent swimming performance in international and Olympic competition. Swimming especially has been the subject of considerable research, much of it focused on conditioning.[5] In the United States much of the

technique and training programs have stemmed from the work of J. E. "Doc" Counsilman, the legendary swimming coach of Indiana University.[3] Some observers believe that swimming records may be approaching a "stall" point since so much efficiency and power have been attained through stroke mechanics and training. Another significant factor in U.S. success in swimming is its age-group programs.[8] No other group of young sports athletes undergo training of the intensity and magnitude of age-group swimmers. A carefully controlled program early may enhance ultimate performance, but it would be extremely difficult to study such a proposal.

The terms off-season, pre-season, and in-season may sound foreign to some swimmers and swimming coaches. For many swimmers, conditioning goes on literally year round, but there is usually a shift in the emphasis and intensity of conditioning from one portion of the year to another. Conditioning intensity increases from off-season, to pre-season, to in-season, reaching its peak in the latter stages of the in-season. Swim coaches and swimmers also use the "taper" just prior to the major event. The taper, or reduction in training intensity or distance, is used because of the extreme overdistance practiced by many swimmers. Swimming has the added unique factor that the conditioning mode must be specific to swimming. This requires year-round access to a swimming pool. Conditioning in water enables the swimmer to spend many more hours in training. (Many elite swimmers cover more than 20,000m daily.) The swimmer does not have to contend with the trauma to the joints experienced by the runner. The cool medium of the pool also enables the swimmer to work at higher percentages of max capacity with less body heat buildup compared to runners.[5] Basically, swimming performances can be clustered into two groups: 1) sprint swimming, and 2) intermediate and long-distance swimming.

SPRINT AND DISTANCE SWIMMING

Sprint Swimming

Major performance factors in sprint swimming are speed, acceleration, and arm power. These performances rely entirely upon *anaerobic* (Stage I, ATP–CP) energy sources. A maximum burst of effort is needed to begin the event and it can be performed with a minimum of breathing because of its brevity. Stored ATP is sufficient to fuel the energy requirements of very short sprints (50 meters, 25-30 seconds). In the 100m sprint swim, the athlete is also making use of *anaerobic* (Stage II, AN–LA) energy sources. That effort, similar to the 440-yard run in track, produces the maximum oxygen debt. The details of that mechanism are described in Chapter 2. The 200m swim engages both Stage II and Stage III and is approximately 60 percent anaerobic and 40 percent aerobic. Bonner[2] has carefully analyzed the energy systems used in swimming.

Strength and power are major factors in sprint swimming. Arm power is a crucial factor in sprints, just as is leg power. Strength requirements are greater in swimming than in running because of the need to move the limbs rapidly and forcefully through the resistance of the water. Sharp and Costill[7] have recently found that increases in sprint speed were associated with increases in power regardless of the strength training device used. This suggests that power, which is best developed through high speed and repetitions at reduced resistance, may be the major focus of future training in swimming as well as in other sports.[6]

Intermediate and Long-Distance Swimming

Long-distance swimming is a maximum challenge of *aerobic* power. Swimming in the range of 200m to 500m requires a mixture of *anaerobic* and *aerobic* performance. The amount of energy drawn from aerobic sources increases from 200m to 500m, while the amount of energy supplied by anaerobic resources during those distances de-

creases. These swimming events are excellent examples of the need to train slow-twitch (red) aerobic fibers as well as fast-twitch (white) anaerobic fibers. Only a few other sporting events require the intense training of both types of fibers that intermediate distance swimming requires. Running in the range of one-half mile to two miles is similar.

Strength training for distance and intermediate swimmers is predominately high-repetition, fast-speed, low-resistance training. The objective is to increase primarily local muscular endurance and, to a lesser degree, muscular strength. Resistance of the water, even at slower swimming speeds, does require development of muscular strength.

Every effort should be made to train aerobically and anaerobically if both energy systems are required by a particular event. If an activity requires 50 percent aerobic energy and 50 percent anaerobic energy, then the training regimen should match the energy requirements of the task. It has been found that strength can be developed in a wide range of sets and repetitions. Like strength, aerobic or anaerobic power can also be developed through a wide range of sets and repetitions of either aerobic or anaerobic conditioning. This suggests that there is no one best combination of sets and repetitions for producing maximum aerobic or anaerobic power. The guideline intervals listed in Figure 3.4 are intended to be just that—guidelines. Precise intensity and duration of aerobic or anaerobic training must be determined by the capacity of the individual athlete. Eynon and Thoden[4] have completed a lengthy review of the science and art of training for competitive swimming. They concur with the view of the authors that the application of more specificity in training would significantly increase the efficiency of conditioning programs. The "season training plan" is similar in objectives to the year-round conditioning approach proposed by the authors.

OFF-SEASON

The major objectives of the off-season conditioning program for sprint swimmers are to increase strength and arm power, and to maintain anaerobic swimming power. Strength training is designed to meet the first objectives, and anaerobic conditioning of a reduced intensity is designed to meet

Warm-Up and Stretching

Anaerobic Conditioning (sprint swimmers)

	Distance	% Max.	Rest	Reps
Swim: (alternate sessions)	50 yds.	75–85%	1 min.	10
	100 yds.	75–85%	2 mins.	10

Aerobic Conditioning (intermediate and long-distance swimmers)

Intermediate Distance

	Distance	% Max.	Rest	Reps
Swim: (alternate sessions)	200 yds.	75%↑	3 mins.	4–6
	800 yds.	75%	—	1

Long Distance

	Distance	% Max.	Rest	Reps
Swim: (alternate sessions)	1500–3000 yds.	75%	—	1
	200 yds.	75%↑	3 mins.	4–6

Strength Training—Train Explosively!

Monday & Friday

Bench Press
6–10 sets, 10-10-8-8-6-6-4-4

Half-Squat
6–10 sets, 8-8-8-8-6-6-4-4

Lateral Raises
5 sets, 10–15 reps

Sit-Ups and/or Leg Lifts
5 sets, 10–25 reps

Tricep Pushdown
5 sets, 8–10 reps

Hyperextension
5 sets, 10 reps

Leg Curl
5 sets, 10–15 reps

Upright Rowing
5 sets, 10 reps

Bent Arm Pullover
5 sets, 10 reps

Bent Over Rowing (with dumbbells)
5 sets, 10 reps

Wednesday

Military Press
6–8 sets, 10-10-8-8-6-6

Jumping Squat
5 sets, 8–15 reps

Clean
5 sets, 8-6-5-4-3

Sit-Ups and/or Leg Lifts
5 sets, 10–25 reps

Tricep Pushdown
5 sets, 8–10 reps

Hyperextension
5 sets, 10 reps

Leg Curl
5 sets, 10–15 reps

Upright Rowing
5 sets, 10 reps

Bent Arm Pullover
5 sets, 10 reps

Bent Over Rowing (with dumbbells)
5 sets, 10 reps

Specialty Exercises

Backstroke

Backstroke Motion (with pulley)
5 sets, 10 reps

Kicking Motion (with ankle weights)
5 sets, 10–50 reps

Butterfly

Butterfly Power Movement (prone with pulley)
5 sets, 10 reps

Arm Rotators (withd umbbells or pulleys)
5 sets, 8–15 reps

FIGURE 15.1 *Off-Season Conditioning Program for Swimming*

Breaststroke

Breaststroke Motion (prone, with pulley)
5 sets, 10 reps

Kicking Motion
5 sets, 10–25 reps

Arm Rotators

Freestyle

Crawl Stroke Arm Motion (prone with pulley)
5 sets, 10 reps

Kicking Motion (with ankle weights)
5 sets, 10–50 reps

Arm Rotators (with dumbbells or pulleys)
5 sets, 8–15 reps

Optional Exercises

Hyperextension, Behind Neck Press, Bar Dips, Incline Press, Frontal Deltoid Raises, Toe Raises.

Stretching Exercises

FIGURE 15.1 *(Continued)*

the latter. Since anaerobic performance in the lactic acid energy range is so intense and fatiguing, the swimmer must be cautioned not to overtrain during the off-season.

Off-season conditioning for intermediate and long-distance swimming is designed primarily to help the athlete maintain aerobic power and strength. Aerobic conditioning will not be as intense as it will be later in the pre-season and in-season periods. Strength training is designed primarily to increase local muscular endurance and, to a lesser degree, strength. The endurance swimmer should always do many repetitions with less resistance in strength training in order to develop muscular endurance. Like the sprint swimmer, the distance swimmer piles up many thousands of yards in training and must be cautious not to train too intensely during off-season. Probably no other athletes train as long and consistently during the off-season as endurance swimmers and runners.

An off-season conditioning program for swimming is offered in Figure 15.1.

The flexibility and stretching program for swimmers, like other athletes, should follow a consistent, year-round maintenance approach.[1]

PRE-SEASON AND IN-SEASON

In the pre-season period, training for anaerobic development intensifies for sprint swimmers. At this point in the training season, programs must be individualized by coaches and athletes. The programs offered here can serve only as a general guide because some athletes may be capable of much greater amounts of work, while others may struggle

to maintain the recommended programs. Strength training for the sprint swimmer will taper off during the pre-season and in-season periods. At the same time, anaerobic conditioning will increase in both amount and intensity. Strength training should be done at high speed with low resistance during these periods. Since some athletes will be capable of tolerating tremendous amounts of anaerobic interval work, both coaches and athletes must use care to avoid staleness in the latter stages of the competitive season. (See Chapter 8.)

For the long-distance swimmer, the pre-season and in-season training periods will show a gradual increase in the amount and intensity of aerobic training. Middle-distance swimmers will increase both anaerobic and aerobic conditioning. More emphasis will be placed on the anaerobic portion of the middle-distance swimmer's training regimen toward the latter stages of the in-season. As with sprint swimmers, the training program becomes increasingly individualized in the pre-season and in-season periods. The basic objectives of training during these periods will be the same, regardless of the capabilities of the individual swimmer. Through the use of interval training techniques, or continuous training, some swimmers will be capable of covering between fifteen and forty miles of training distance per week as they begin to peak.

In-season strength training for swimmers is minimal. It is designed primarily to maintain strength and should be done not more than once or twice per week. The emphasis is always on high-repetition, fast-speed, and low-resistance exercise. Pre-season and in-season conditioning programs for swimmers are offered in Figures 15.2 and 15.3.

Warm-Up and Stretching

Anaerobic Conditioning (daily)—Sprint Swimmers

	Distance	% Max.	Rest	Reps
	100 yds.	85–95%	2 mins.	10
Swim: (alternate sessions)	50 yds.	85–95%	1 min.	10

Aerobic Conditioning (daily)—Intermediate- and Long-Distance Swimmers

Intermediate Distance

	Distance	% Max.	Rest	Reps
Swim: (alternate sessions)	100 yds.	85–95%	3 mins.	8–12
	200 yds.	85–95%	3 mins.	4–6

Long Distance

	Distance	% Max.	Rest	Reps
Swim: (alternate sessions)	1500–3000 yds.	85–95%	—	1
	200 yds.	85–95%	3 mins.	4–6

Strength Training—Train Explosively!

Monday-Wednesday-Friday

Bench Press
3–5 sets, 10–15 reps

Jumping Squat
3–5 sets, 10–15 reps

Bent Over Row (with dumbbells)
3–5 sets, 10–15 reps

Sit-Ups and/or Leg Lifts
3–5 sets, 10–50 reps

Tricep Pushdown
3–5 sets, 10–20 reps

Hyperextension
3–5 sets, 10–25 reps

Leg Extension
3–5 sets, 10–20 reps

Leg Curl
3–5 sets, 10–20 reps

Upright Rowing
3–5 sets, 10–50 reps

Lateral Raises
3–5 sets, 10–50 reps

Bent Arm Pullover
3–5 sets, 10–15 reps

Specialty Exercises

A. Imitative stroke motion (with pulley) for backstroke, breaststroke, butterfly, or freestyle
B. Imitative kicking motion for various kicks
C. Arm rotators (with dumbbells or pulleys)

Optional Exercises

Hyperextension, Behind Neck Press, Bar Dips, Incline Press, Frontal Deltoid Raises, Toe Raises.

Stretching Exercises

FIGURE 15.2 *Pre-Season Conditioning Program for Swimming*

Warm-Up and Stretching

Anaerobic Conditioning (daily)—Sprint Swimmers

	Distance	% Max.	Rest	Reps	Sets
Swim: (alternate sessions)	50 yds.	95%↑	1 min.	10	1
	25 yds.	100%	30 secs.	10–15	1–2

FIGURE 15.3 *In-Season Conditioning Program for Swimming*

(Continued)

Aerobic Conditioning (daily)—Intermediate- and Long-Distance Swimmers

Intermediate Distance

	Distance	% Max.	Rest	Reps
Swim: (alternate sessions)	50 yds.	100%	1 min.	12–16
	100 yds.	95%↑	3 mins.	8–12
	200 yds.	95%	3 mins.	4–6

Long Distance

	Distance	% Max.	Rest	Reps
Swim: (alternate sessions)	3000–6000 yds.	LSD	—	1
	1500–3000 yds.	95%	—	1
	200 yds.	95%↑	3 mins.	4–6

Strength Training—Train Explosively!

Monday & Wednesday

Jumping Squat 2–3 sets, 10–20 reps	Bench Press, Military Press, or Incline Press 2–5 sets, 10–20 reps	Sit-Ups 2–3 sets, 10–50 reps

Specialty Exercises

A. Imitative stroke motion (with pulley) for backstroke, breaststroke, butterfly, or freestyle
B. Imitative kicking motion for various kicks
C. Arm rotators (with dumbbells or pulleys)

Optional Exercises

Hyperextension, Behind Neck Press, Bar Dips, Incline Press, Frontal Deltoid Raises, Toe Raises.

Stretching Exercises

FIGURE 15.3 *(Continued)*

SPECIALTY EXERCISES

Butterfly, Backstroke, Freestyle, and Breaststroke Motion (with pulley)

These exercises are done by lying on a bench and performing the exact range of motion of the stroke with two wall pulleys. A "Y" attachment may be used if only one pulley is available.

Kicks

The various kicking motions can be performed by supporting the upper body and hips on a bench and imitating the particular kicking motion. Ankle weights, weighted boots, or no weight at all usually works better than a pulley.

Arm Rotators

This exercise is done by rotating the forearm around the elbow, which is used as a pivotal point. Both dumbbells and wall pulleys are effective.

SUMMARY

Swimming involves all three stages of metabolism, individually or in varying combinations according to the event. The sprint events are anaerobic, involving both Stage I or II, while the middle-distance and long-distance events are predominately aerobic. Some intermediate events may mix Stage II (AN–LA) and Stage III (AER). Strength and flexibility are also required for swim events, and power is needed to overcome the resistance of the water.

This chapter contains year-round conditioning

programs aimed at developing the appropriate performance factors for the event. The off-season, pre-season, and in-season programs are intended to be event-specific.

REFERENCES

1. Anderson, Bob. "Stretching for Swimming." *NSCA Journal* 3 (1981): 20–23.
2. Bonner, Hugh W. "Energy Systems used During Swimming." *Swimming Technique* 17 (1980): 10–13.
3. Counsilman, James E. *The Complete Book of Swimming.* New York: Atheneum, 1977.
4. Eynon, Robert, and Thoden, James. "Competitive Swimming. In *The Scientific Aspects of Sports Training*, A. W. Taylor, ed. Springfield, IL: Charles C. Thomas, 1975, pp. 269–290.
5. Faulkner, John A. *What Research Tells the Coach About Swimming.* Washington, D.C.: AAHPER (1976).
6. Jopke, Terry. "Training Swimmers: How Coaches Get Results." *The Physician and Sportsmedicine* 10 (1982): 161–165.
7. Sharp, R. L., and Costill, David L. "Force, Work, and Power: What They Mean to the Competitive Swimmer." *Swimming World* 23 (1982): 41–43.
8. Zauner, Chrintian W. "Training the Child Swimmer." In *Toward an Understanding of Human Performance*, Edmund J. Burke, ed. 2d ed. Ithaca, NY: Mouvement Publications, 1980, pp. 76–77.

16

Track and Field

This chapter contains year-round conditioning programs for track and field. The programs are designed for the off-season, pre-season, and in-season periods. In order to make the most effective use of the programs offered here, the reader is referred to Chapter 3 for the basis of aerobic and anaerobic training programs, to Chapter 4 for the basis of strength programs, to Chapter 5 for the basis of warm-up, stretching, and flexibility programs, and to Chapter 8 for the most efficient means of incorporating those objectives into a single workout. The reader is also referred to the sample recording charts offered in the Appendix. These charts will facilitate the measurement of the athlete's progress in the training program and will indicate the athlete's standing in regard to training goals.

Track and field, as well as swimming, are unique compared to the other team sports listed in Part II. The two areas represent the epitome of aerobic, anaerobic, and in some cases strength and power performances. Conditioning is a major aspect of preparation for both track and field and swimming. Entire books have been written on training and conditioning for both sports. Track events are probably the most thoroughly researched sports activities discussed in this book.[2,5] The authors could not, within limitations of a single chapter, expect to lay out a day-by-day, week-by-week conditioning program for either track or swimming. They have, however, attempted to develop a basic and cohesive year-round conditioning program.

The terms *off-season*, *pre-season*, and *in-season* may sound foreign to some track athletes and coaches. In some events, conditioning literally goes on year round, but there is usually a shift in the emphasis and intensity of conditioning from one

portion of the year to another. Conditioning intensity increases from off-season, to pre-season, to in-season, reaching its peak in the latter stages of the in-season. Because of the distinct differences in the various track and field events, the authors have clustered track and field performances into four basic groups: 1) sprints and hurdles, 2) long-and intermediate-distance running, 3) jumping events, and 4) throwing events.

SPRINTS AND HURDLES

The major performance factors in short (50m–100m) sprint races and hurdles are speed, acceleration, and leg power. These performances rely entirely on *anaerobic* (ATP-CP) energy sources. There is a maximum burst of effort and the event can literally be performed without breathing because it is so brief. Stored ATP is sufficient to fuel the energy requirements of short sprints and hurdles. In sprint races between 200m and 400m, the athlete is also making use of *anaerobic* Stage II (AN–LA) energy sources. The 400m event produces the maximum oxygen debt, the details of which are described in Chapter 2. While acceleration and leg power as well as speed are the major factors in the short sprints, anaerobic capacity becomes increasingly important beyond 80m, as readily available ATP is exhausted.[5]

Dintiman[5] has made a major review of sprinting research. He has made several important generalizations: 1) Increased strength leads to an increase in the speed of muscle contraction; 2) more recent work has found a significant correlation between lower body strength and speed in sprinting; and 3) a program of flexibility training, strength training, and sprinting resulted in the best 40-yd.

speed and was significantly better than sprinting only. Supplemental training must be conducted *in addition* to sprinting practice to be effective.

Off-Season

The major objectives of the off-season conditioning program for sprinters and hurdlers are to increase strength and leg power, and to maintain anaerobic running speed. Strength training is designed to meet the first objectives, and anaerobic conditioning of reduced intensity is designed to meet the latter. Since anaerobic performance in the lactic acid energy range is so tense and fa-

tiguing, the athlete must be cautioned not to overtrain during the off-season. Off-season programs for sprinters and hurdlers are offered in Figures 16.1 and 16.2.

Pre-Season and In-Season

In the pre-season period, training for anaerobic development intensifies for sprinters and hurdlers. At this point in the training season programs must be individualized by coaches or athletes. The programs offered here can serve only as a general guide because some athletes will be capable of much greater amounts of work, while others may

---

Warm-Up and Stretching

Anaerobic Conditioning

Shorter Sprints

	Distance	% Max.	Rest	Reps
Run: (alternate days)	100 yds.	75–85%	1 min.	10
	220 yds.	75–85%	2 mins.	10

Longer Sprints

	Distance	% Max.	Rest	Reps
Run: (alternate days)	440 yds.	75–85%	3–5 mins.	10
	880 yds.	75–85%	3–5 mins.	10

Strength Training—Train Explosively!

Monday & Friday

Bench Press 10-10-8-8-8-8-6-6	Leg Thrust 5 sets, 10 reps
Half-Squat 10-10-8-8-8-8-6-6	Leg Curl (toes in) 5 sets, 10–15 reps
Good Morning 5 sets, 10 reps	Toe Raises 8 sets, 30 reps

Wednesday

Incline Press 6 sets, 8-8-6-6-6-6	Leg Curl (toes in) 5 sets, 10–15 reps
High Pull 8-6-5-5-5	High Knee Lift 3 sets, 10 reps
Leg Thrust 5 sets, 10 reps	Toe Raises 8 sets, 30 reps

Optional Exercises

Leg Extension, Bent Arm Pullover, Lat Pull, Upright Rowing, Running Motion (with dumbbells), Bar Dips.

Stretching Exercises

FIGURE 16.1 *Off-Season Conditioning Program for Sprints*

Warm-Up and Stretching

Anaerobic Conditioning

Shorter Hurdles

	Distance	% Max.	Rest	Reps
Run: (alternate days)	100 yds.	75–85%	1 min.	10
	220 yds.	75–85%	2 mins.	10

Longer Hurdles

	Distance	% Max.	Rest	Reps
Run: (alternate days)	440 yds.	75–85%	3–5 mins.	10
	880 yds.	75–85%	3–5 mins.	10

Strength Training—Train Explosively!

Monday & Friday

Incline Press
2 weeks of 10-10-8-8-8-8-8-8
2 weeks of 8-8-8-8-6-6-6-6

Bent Over Rowing
6 sets, 10 reps

Half Squat
4 weeks of 8-8-8-8-8-8-6-6
4 weeks of 8-8-8-8-6-6-6-6

Leg Curl
5 sets, 10 reps

Toe Raises
8 sets, 30 reps

High Knee Lift
3–5 sets, 10 reps

Trailing Leg Exercise
5 sets, 10 reps

Sit-Ups (twisting)
5 sets, 10–15 reps

Leg Thrust
5 sets, 10 reps

Wednesday

Bench Press
10-10-8-8-8-8

High Pull
8-6-5-5-5

Incline Flys
5 sets, 10 reps

Toe Raises
8 sets, 30 reps

Leg Thrust
5 sets, 10 reps

Lat Pulls
6 sets, 10 reps

Leg Curl
5 sets, 10 reps

Sit-Ups (twisting)
5 sets, 10 reps

High Knee Lift
5 sets, 10 reps

Stretching Exercises

FIGURE 16.2 *Off-Season Conditioning Program for Hurdles*

struggle to maintain the recommended programs. Strength training will taper off during the pre-season and into the in-season period, while anaerobic conditioning will increase both in amount and intensity. Strength training should be done at high speed with low resistance during these periods. Since some athletes will be capable of tolerating tremendous amounts of (anaerobic) interval work, both coaches and athletes must use care to avoid staleness in the latter stages of the competitive season. (See Chapter 8.)

Pre-season and in-season conditioning programs for sprinting and hurdling are offered in Figures 16.3, 16.4, 16.5, and 16.6.

Warm-Up and Stretching

Anaerobic Conditioning

Shorter Sprints

	Distance	% Max.	Rest	Reps	Sets
Run: (M-W-F)	100 yds.	85–95%	1 min.	10	1
	220 yds.	85–95%	2 mins.	10	1

Longer Sprints

	Distance	% Max.	Rest	Reps	Sets
Run: (M-W-F)	440 yds.	85–95%	3 mins.	10	1
	880 yds.	85–95%	3 mins.	10	1

Strength Training—Train Explosively!

Monday-Wednesday-Friday

Bench Press
3–6 sets, 10–15 reps

Jumping Squat
3–5 sets, 10–15 reps

High Knee Lift
3–5 sets, 10 reps

Leg Curl
3–5 sets, 10–15 reps

Good Morning
3–5 sets, 10–15 reps

Leg Thrust
3–5 sets, 10–15 reps

Toe Raises
3–5 sets, 30–75 reps

Sit-Ups
3–5 sets, 10–50 reps

Stretching Exercises

FIGURE 16.3   *Pre-Season Conditioning Program for Sprints*

Warm-Up and Stretching

Anaerobic Conditioning

Shorter Hurdles

	Distance	% Max.	Rest	Reps	Sets
Run: (M-W-F)	100 yds.	85–95%	1 min.	10	1
	220 yds.	85–95%	2 mins.	10	1

Longer Hurdles

	Distance	% Max.	Rest	Reps	Sets
Run: (M-W-F)	440 yds.	85–95%	3 mins.	10	1
	880 yds.	85–95%	3 mins.	10	1

Strength Training—Train Explosively!

Monday & Friday

Incline Press
3–6 sets, 6–12 reps

Bent Over Rowing
3–5 sets, 10–15

Wednesday

Bench Press
3–6 sets, 6–12 reps

*Incline Flys
3–5 sets, 10–15 reps

*Light weight, high reps, fast speed

FIGURE 16.4   *Pre-season Conditioning Program for Hurdles*

(Continued)

Monday & Friday	*Wednesday*
*Jumping Squat 3–5 sets, 10–15 reps	High Pull 3–5 sets, 8-6-5-5-3
*Toe Raises 3–5 sets, 30–75 reps	*Toe Raises 3–5 sets, 30–75 reps
*Trailing Leg Exercise 3–5 sets, 8–15 reps	*Trailing Leg Exercise 3–5 sets, 8–15 reps
*High Knee Lift 3–5 sets, 8–15 reps	*High Knee Lift 3–5 sets, 8–15 reps
*Leg Thrust 3–5 sets, 8–15 reps	*Leg Thrust 3–5 sets, 8–15 reps
*Leg Curl 3–5 sets, 8–15 reps	*Leg Curl 3–5 sets, 8–15 reps
Sit-Ups (twisting) 3–5 sets, 10–50 reps	Sit-Ups (twisting) 3–5 sets, 10–50 reps
Stretching Exercises	*Stretching Exercises*
*Light weight, high reps, fast speed	

FIGURE 16.4 *(Continued)*

Warm-Up and Stretching

Anaerobic Training (daily)

Shorter Sprints

	Distance	% Max.	Rest	Reps	Sets
Run: (daily)	100 yds.	95%↑	1 min.	10	1
	50 yds.	100%	30 secs.	10–15	2

Longer Sprints

	Distance	% Max.	Rest	Reps	Sets
Run: (daily)	220 yds.	95%↑	3 mins.	10–15	1
	440 yds.	90–95%	3 mins.	8–10	1

Strength Training—Train Explosively!

Monday & Wednesday

*Running Motion (with dumbbells)
2–3 sets, 15–25 reps

Any or All Speed Exercises
High Knee Lift, Leg Curl (toes in),
Leg Thrust. Select any combination.

Bench Press or Bent Arm Pullover
2–3 sets, 10–15 reps

Optional Exercises
Leg Extension, Bent Arm Pullover, Lat Pull, Upright Rowing, Bar Dips.

Stretching Exercises

*Light weight, high reps, fast speed

FIGURE 16.5 *In-Season Conditioning Program for Sprints*

Warm-Up and Stretching

Anaerobic Conditioning (daily)

Shorter Hurdles

	Distance	% Max.	Rest	Reps	Sets
Run: (daily)	100 yds.	95%↑	1 min.	10	1
	50 yds.	100%	30 secs.	10–15	2

Longer Hurdles

	Distance	% Max.	Rest	Reps	Sets
Run: (daily)	220 yds.	95%↑	3 mins.	10–15	1
	440 yds.	90–95%	3 mins.	8–10	1

Strength Training—Train Explosively!

Monday & Wednesday

Bench Press
2–3 sets, 10–15 reps

Jumping Squats
2–3 sets, 10–15 reps

Running Motion (with dumbbells)
2–3 sets, 15–25 reps

Speed Exercises
High Knee Lift, Leg Curl (toes in).
Select any combination of these.

Trailing Leg Exercise
2–3 sets, 10–15 reps

Stretching Exercises

FIGURE 16.6 *In-Season Conditioning Program for Hurdles*

LONG- AND INTERMEDIATE-DISTANCE RUNNING

Much of the basis for both anaerobic and aerobic running has been discussed in Chapter 3, Aerobic and Anaerobic Conditioning. It is no surprise that elite distance runners are among the greatest aerobic athletes with maximal oxygen uptakes in the range of 70-80 ml/kg of body weight.[2] This exceeds the range for elite endurance swimmers.

Long-distance running has also been the subject of a tremendous amount of research. There are several excellent scientific reviews of the topic of distance running.[2, 3, 4, 10] Much of the research on distance running has focused on the need to accomplish long-slow-distance training versus the need to develop speed through shorter and more intense intervals. Costill[2] has concluded that both speed (interval) and overdistance work are necessary for maximum training effect and performance. Daniels et al.[4] maintain that there is no all-encompassing training routine for distance runners and that programs must be individualized to meet specific strengths and weaknesses.

Long-distance running is the ultimate challenge of *aerobic* power. The marathon run is the greatest competitive endurance feat. Running in the range of one-half mile to two miles requires a mixture of anaerobic and aerobic performance. The amount of energy drawn from aerobic sources increases during the distance from one-half mile to two miles, while the amount of energy supplied by anaerobic resources during that distance decreases. These events provide an excellent example of the need to train slow-twitch (red) aerobic fibers as well as fast-twitch (white) anaerobic fibers. Only a few other sporting events require the kind of intense training of both types of fibers that inter-mediate-distance running requires. Strength training for long- and intermediate-distance runners is predominately high-repetition, low-resistance training. The objective is to increase primarily local muscular endurance and, to a lesser degree, muscular strength.

Every effort should be made to train aerobically and anaerobically if both energy systems are required by a particular event. If an activity requires 50 percent aerobic energy and 50 percent anaerobic energy, then the training regimen should match the energy requirements of the task. Strength can be developed in a wide range of sets and repetitions of either aerobic or anaerobic conditioning. This suggests that there is no one best combination of sets and repetitions for producing maximum aerobic or anaerobic power. The guideline intervals listed in Figure 3.4 are intended to be just that—guidelines. The precise intensity and duration of aerobic or anaerobic training must be determined by the capacity of the athlete.

Distance running is particularly conducive to the tightening of muscles and a loss of flexibility. A year-round stretching and flexibility program should be part of the preparation for intermediate and long-distance runners[1]. Once a program has been established, it should be followed year round on a maintenance schedule.

Off-Season

Off-season conditioning for long- and intermediate-distance running is designed primarily to maintain aerobic power. Aerobic training will not be as intense as it will be later in the pre-season and in-season periods. Strength training is designed primarily to increase local muscular endurance and, to a lesser degree, increase strength. This means that the endurance athlete will always do many repetitions with less resistance in strength training. Like the sprinter, the distance runner piles up many miles in training and must be cautious not to train too intensely during the off-season. Per-

---

Warm-Up and Stretching

Aerobic Conditioning

Intermediate-Distance Runners

	Distance	% Max.	Rest	Reps
Run: (alternate days)	880 yds.	75%↑	3 mins.	4–6
	2 mi.	75%↑	—	1

Long-Distance Runners

	Distance	% Max.	Rest	Reps
Run: (alternate days)	3–5 mi.	75%	—	1
	880 yds.	75%↑	3 mins.	4–6

Strength Training—Train Explosively

Monday & Friday

Bench Press
6 sets, 15–20 reps

Upright Rowing
6 sets, 15–20 reps

Curls (with dumbbells)
6 sets, 10–20 reps

Good Morning
6 sets, 10–20 reps

Half-Squat
8 sets, 10-10-10-10-8-8-8-8

Sit Ups (twisting)
6 sets, 15–20 reps

Toe Raises
8 sets, 30–50 reps

Wednesday

Bench (with dumbbells)
6 sets, 15–20 reps

High Pull
8-8-6-6-5

Curls (with dumbbells)
6 sets, 10–20 reps

Good Morning
6 sets, 10–20 reps

Sit-Ups (twisting)
6 sets, 15–20 reps

Toe Raises
8 sets, 30–50 reps

Optional Exercises

Running Motion (with dumbbells), Lat Pulls, Bent Over Rowing, Leg Extension, Upright Rowing, High Knee Lift.

Stretching Exercises

FIGURE 16.7 *Off-Season Conditioning Program for Long- and Intermediate-Distance Running* haps no other athletes train as long and consistently during the off-season as endurance runners and swimmers.

An off-season conditioning program for long- and intermediate-distance runners is offered in Figure 16.7.

Pre-Season and In-Season

In the pre-season and in-season training periods there is a gradual increase in the amount and intensity of aerobic training for distance runners. Middle-distance runners should increase the amounts of both anaerobic and aerobic conditioning. More emphasis should be placed on the anaerobic portion of the middle-distance runner's training regimen toward the latter stages of the in-season. As with sprinters, the training program becomes increasingly individualized during the pre-season and in-season periods. The basic objectives of training during these periods will be the same, regardless of the capabilities of the individual runner. Through the use of continuous training or aerobic intervals, some distance runners will be capable of covering between 100 and 200 miles of training distance per week as they begin to peak.

In-season strength training for intermediate- and long-distance runners is very minimal. It is designed primarily to maintain strength and should not be done more than once or twice per week. Strength training for these athletes is always high-repetition, fast-speed, and low-resistance exercise.

Pre-season and in-season conditioning programs are offered in Figures 16.8 and 16.9.

Warm-Up and Stretching

Aerobic-Anaerobic Conditioning (daily)

Intermediate-Distance Runners

	Distance	% Max.	Rest	Reps
Run: (alternate days)	440 yds.	85–95%	3 mins.	8–12
	880 yds.	85–95%	3 mins.	4–6

Long-Distance Runners

	Distance	% Max.	Rest	Reps
Run: (alternate days)	3–5 mi.	85–95%	—	1
	880 yds.	85–95%	3 mins.	4–6

Strength Training—Train Explosively!

Monday & Friday

Bench Press
3–5 sets, 8–15 reps

Upright Rowing
3–5 sets, 10–15 reps

Curls (with dumbbells)
3–5 sets, 10–15 reps

Good Morning
3–5 sets, 10 reps

Jumping Squat
3–5 sets, 8–15 reps

Sit-Ups (twisting)
3–5 sets, 15–50 reps

Toe Raises
3–5 sets, 30–75

Wednesday

Bench Press (with dumbbells)
3–5 sets, 6–10 reps

High Pull
5 sets, 8-5-5-3-3

Curls (with dumbbells)
3–5 sets, 10–15 reps

Good Morning
3–5 sets, 10 reps

Sit-Ups (twisting)
3–5 sets, 15–50 reps

Toe Raises
3–5 sets, 30–75 reps

FIGURE 16.8 *Pre-Season Conditioning Program for Long- and Intermediate-Distance Running*

(Continued)

Optional Exercises

Running Motion (with dumbbells), Lat Pulls, Bent Over Rowing, Leg Extension, Upright Rowing, High Knee Lift.

Stretching Exercises

FIGURE 16.8 *(Continued)*

Warm-Up and Stretching

Aerobic-Anaerobic Conditioning (daily)

Intermediate-Distance Runners

	Distance	*% Max.*	*Rest*	*Reps*
Run: (alternate days)	220 yds.	100%	1 min.	12–16
	440 yds.	95%↑	3 mins.	8–12
	880 yds.	95%	3 mins.	4–6

Long-Distance Runners

	Distance	*% Max.*	*Rest*	*Reps*
Run: (alternate days)	5–10 mi.	LSD	—	1
	3–5 mi.	95%↑	—	1
	880 yds.	95%↑	3 mins.	4–6

Strength Training—Train Explosively!
 (1–2 per week)

Bench Press
2–3 sets, 10–25 reps

Jumping Squat
2–3 sets, 10–20 reps

Curls (with dumbbells)
2–3 sets, 10–15 reps

Optional Exercises

High Knee Lift, Running Motion (with dumbbells), Toe Raises, Sit-Ups, Hyperextension or Good Mornings.

Stretching Exercises

FIGURE 16.9 *In-Season Conditioning Program for Long- and Intermediate-Distance Runners*

JUMPING EVENTS

Jumping events rely primarily upon leg power, acceleration, and, in three of the four jumping events, running speed. Strength training is a very significant factor in year-round conditioning for jumping events. Strength training is used to increase leg power for the high jumper, arm and upper body strength for the pole vaulter, and acceleration for the long jumper. The Soviets have evolved extensive progressive resistance programs for developing strength and explosive power.[7] They utilize a variety of weights and techniques from heavy resistance squats to high speed jumps with light weights. They also use depth jumps and as many as 1200-1300 practice jumps per year.

Anaerobic sprints should comprise a major portion of the conditioning for long jumpers and triple jumpers. Speed development as indicated is extremely important for jumpers. *Flexibility* is also especially important to the pole vaulter and high jumper. Year-round conditioning programs for high jumpers and long jumpers are offered in Figures 16.10, 16.11, and 16.12.

THROWING EVENTS

Throwing in field events relies primarily upon *power* and *strength*, and thus strength training is the essential supplementary conditioning tech-nique. Athletes in the throwing events were among the first to make significant use of weight training to improve their athletic performance. Parry O'Brien was a pioneer in the use of weight train-ing as a supplement to his shot-putting preparation in the 1950s. He reported a corresponding increase in putting the shot with systematic increases in strength. Just as the endurance athlete focuses almost entirely upon aerobic conditioning, the throwing event athlete focuses almost entirely upon strength training. The general principles of

---

Warm-Up and Stretching

Strength Training—Train Explosively!

Monday & Friday	*Wednesday*
Bench Press	Military Press or Incline Press
6–8 sets, 10-10-8-8-6-6-4-4	6–8 sets, 10-10-8-8-6-6-4-4
Half-Squat	Jumping Squats
6–8 sets, 8-8-8-8-6-6-4-4	6–8 sets, 10 reps
Toe Raises	Toe Raises
6–8 sets, 30–75 reps	6–8 sets, 30–75 reps
Cleans	Cleans
5 sets, 8-5-5-3-3	5 sets, 8-5-5-3-3
High Knee Lift	High Knee Lift
5 sets, 10 reps	5 sets, 10 reps
Leg Curl (toes in)	Leg Curl (toes in)
5 sets, 10 reps	5 sets, 10 reps
Sit-Ups and/or Leg Lifts	Sit-Ups and/or Leg Lifts
5 sets, 10–20 reps	5 sets, 10–20 reps

Optional Exercises

Running Arm Motion (with dumbbells), Bar Dips, Lat Pulls, Bent Over Rowing, Rack Squat, Leg Extension, Curls, Upright Rowing, Good Morning, Frontal Delts.

Specialty Exercises

High Jump	*Pole Vault*	*Triple Jump*	*Long Jump*
High Jump Leg Motion	Bent Arm Pullover	High Rack Squat	Ankle Exercise
5 sets, 10 reps	5 sets, 10 reps	5 sets, 5-5-3-3-1	3–5 sets, 15 reps
	Pull-Ups	Step-Ups	
	3–5 sets	3–5 sets, 5–10 reps	
	Grip Exercises		
	3–5 sets		

Anaerobic Conditioning

		Distance	*% Max.*	*Rest*	*Reps*
	Run:	100 yds.	85–95%	1 min.	8–10

Stretching Exercises

FIGURE 16.10   *Off-Season Conditioning Program for High Jump, Pole Vault, Triple Jump, and Long Jump*

Warm-Up and Stretching

Strength Training—Train Explosively!

Monday-Wednesday-Friday

Bench Press 3–6 sets, 10–20 reps	High Knee Lift 5 sets, 10–15 reps
Half-Squat 3–6 sets, 10–20 reps	Leg Curls (toes in) 5 sets, 10–15 reps
Toe Raises 3–6 sets	Sit-Ups and/or Leg Lifts 5 sets, 10–25 reps
Cleans 5 sets, 8-5-5-3-3	

Optional Exercises

Running Arm Motion (with dumbbells), Bar Dips, Lat Pulls, Bent Over Rowing, Rack Squat, Leg Extension, Curls, Upright Rowing, Good Morning, Frontal Delts.

Specialty Exercises

High Jump	*Pole Vault*	*Triple Jump*	*Long Jump*
High Jump Leg Motion 5 sets, 10 reps	Bent Arm Pullover 5 sets, 10 reps	High Rack Squat 5 sets, 5-5-3-3-1	Ankle Exercise 3–5 sets, 15 reps
	Pull-Ups 3–5 sets	Step-Ups 3–5 sets, 5–10 reps	
	Grip Exercises 3–5 sets		

Anaerobic Conditioning

		Distance	% Max.	Rest	Reps
	Run:	100 yds.	95%↑	1 min.	10–12

Stretching Exercises

FIGURE 16.11 *Pre-Season Conditioning Program for High Jump, Pole Vault, Triple Jump, and Long Jump*

Warm-Up and Stretching

Strength Training—Train Explosively!

Monday	*Wednesday*
Bench Press 2–3 sets, 10–15 reps	Military Press 2–3 sets, 10–15 reps
High Knee Lift 2–3 sets, 10–15 reps	High Knee Lift 2–3 sets, 10–15 reps
Jumping Squat 2–3 sets, 12–20 reps	Jumping Squat 2–3 sets, 12–20 reps
Toe Raises 2–3 sets, 30 reps	Toe Raises 2–3 sets, 30 reps

Optional Exercises

Running Arm Motion (with dumbbells), Bar Dips, Lat Pulls, Bent Over Rowing, Rack Squat, Leg Extension, Curls, Upright Rowing, Good Morning, Frontal Delts.

FIGURE 16.12 *In-Season Conditioning Program for High Jump, Pole Vault, Triple Jump, and Long Jump*

(Continued)

Specialty Exercises

High Jump	*Pole Vault*	*Triple Jump*	*Long Jump*
High Jump Leg Motion	Bent Arm Pullover	High Rack Squat	Ankle Exercise
5 sets, 10 reps	5 sets, 10 reps	5 sets, 5-5-3-3-1	3-5 sets, 15 reps
	Pull-Ups	Step-Ups	
	3-5 sets	3-5 sets, 5-10 reps	
	Grip Exercises		
	3-5 sets		

Anaerobic Conditioning (daily)

		Distance	*% Max.*	*Rest*	*Reps*
	Run:	50 yds.	100%	30 secs.	10-15

Stretching Exercises

FIGURE 16.12 *(Continued)*

Monday-Wednesday-Friday

Squat and Bench Press

Preparation Period	*Weeks*	*Rating*	*Weeks*	*Rating*
Preparation Period	1) 15-15-15	L	5) 12-12-10-10	L
	2) 15-15-15	M	6) 10-10-10	M
	3) 15-15-15	MH	7) 10-10-10	MH
	4) 12-12-10-10	H	8) 10-10-10	H
Regular Off-Season	1) 10-10-8-8-6-6	L	9) 8-8-6-6-4-4	L
	2) 10-10-8-8-6-6	M	10) 8-8-6-6-4-4	M
	3) 10-10-8-8-6-6	MH	11) 8-8-6-6-4-4	MH
	4) 10-10-8-8-6-6	H	12) 8-8-6-6-4-4	H
	5) 8-8-6-6-5-5	L	13) 8-8-5-5-3-3	L
	6) 8-8-6-6-5-5	M	14) 8-8-5-5-3-3	M
	7) 8-8-6-6-5-5	MH	15) 8-8-5-5-3-3	MH
	8) 8-8-6-6-5-5	H	16) 8-8-5-5-3-3	H

Power Cleans or High Pulls

Preparation Period	*Weeks*	*Rating*	*Weeks*	*Rating*
Preparation Period	1) 5-5-5-5-5	L	5) 5-5-4-4-4	L
	2) 5-5-5-5-5	M	6) 5-5-4-4-4	M
	3) 5-5-5-5-5	MH	7) 5-4-4-4-3	MH
	4) 5-5-4-4-4	H	8) 5-4-4-3-3	H
Regular Off-Season	1) 5-4-4-4-4	L	9) 5-4-3-3-3	L
	2) 5-4-4-4-4	M	10) 5-4-3-3-3	M
	3) 5-4-4-4-4	MH	11) 5-4-3-3-3	MH
	4) 5-4-4-4-4	H	12) 5-4-3-3-3	H
	5) 5-4-4-3-3	L	13) 5-4-3-2-2	L
	6) 5-4-4-3-3	M	14) 5-4-3-2-2	M
	7) 5-4-4-3-3	MH	15) 5-4-3-2-2	MH
	8) 5-4-4-3-3	H	16) 5-4-3-2-2	H

FIGURE 16.13 *Off-Season Conditioning Program for Shot-Put, Discus, and Javelin*

(Continued)

Supplemental and Specialty Exercises

Bent Arm Laterals***
Preparatory, 5 sets, 8 reps
Regular, 4 sets, 8 reps

Incline Dumbbell Press**
Preparatory, 5 sets, 8 reps
Regular, 4 sets, 8 reps

Bent Arm Pullover
Preparatory, 5 sets, 8 reps
Regular, 5 sets, 8 reps

Leg Extension
Preparatory, 4 sets, 12 reps
Regular, 4 sets, 10 reps

Leg Curl
Preparatory, 4 sets, 12 reps
Regular, 4 sets, 10 reps

Good Morning***, **
Preparatory, 4 sets, 8 reps
Regular, 4 sets, 8 reps

Hyperextension*
Preparatory, 5 sets, 12 reps
Regular, 4 sets, 10 reps

Tricep Pushdown
Preparatory, 4 sets, 10 reps
Regular, 4 sets, 8 reps

Toe Raises
Preparatory, 4 sets, 12 reps
Regular, 4 sets, 10 reps

Wrist Curl
Preparatory, 4 sets, 10 reps
Regular, 4 sets, 10 reps

Optional Exercises
Incline Press, Snatch Pull, Military Press.

***Indicates specialty exercise for discus.
 **Indicates specialty exercise for shot-put.
  *Indicates specialty exercise for javelin.

FIGURE 16.13 *(Continued)*

strength training recommended for all athletes should be followed, and the intensity of training should peak during the in-season period.

The note to train explosively, which appears in every training program in this book, is particularly pertinent to throwing event athletes. These performers are involved in the development of anaerobic, fast-twitch fibers. The ability to make use of the strength developed in training will be determined by the specificity of training. High-speed, explosive movements in strength training are essential for throwing events. Strength training should always be accompanied with event (skill) practice[7]. Although strength is a major factor in throwing events, skill is also an important factor, especially with the hammer throw and the javelin. The discus and shot are more influenced by power, but also utilize skilled movements.

Flexibility is also important in throwing events, since a full range-of-motion is needed to achieve maximum throwing performance[7]. A flexibility program should be followed year round for maximum effectiveness.

For the heavy year-round strength program necessary for the weight events, it is best to utilize a cycle system. (See Chapter 4). The following cycle system has been designed especially for the weight event. To execute the system, follow these guidelines:

1. Find the athlete's 1RM for each major and assistant exercise to be trained.
2. Find the athlete's projected 1RM for the 16-week cycle. Use a 7½ percent increase for athletes in the first or second of heavy strength training, or a 5 percent increase for athletes with more advanced strength training experience.
3. The amount of weight (or the resistance level) to use in the numerous repetition series offered can be determined from the following table and the individual's projected maximum.
4. The resistance levels are applied directly to the final two sets of each repetition series for the "heavy" weeks of the cycle.
5. The next table shows the resistance levels to be

Number of reps	Resistance Level
2	95% of projected max
3	90% of projected max
4	85–87% of projected max
5	80% of projected max
6	75% of projected max
7	72½% of projected max
8	70% of projected max
10	60% of projected max
15	50% of projected max

TABLE 16.1 *Number of Repetitions for Projected Strength Maximum*

employed for the final two sets of each repetition series. This is based on the previously indicated "percent of projected max" for that particular number of repetitions.

6. The warm-up and adjustment sets of each repetition series are found in the standard way described in Chapter 4. Table 4.1 is used to determine the starting weights. The resistance levels of the adjustment sets are determined by spacing the increases shown by the "step like" indicators, equidistant apart. When the exact resistance levels are not possible or preferable,

For athletes who squat over 225 pounds and bench press over 135 pounds

		Lower Body	Pulls and Upper Body
Heavy week	indicated % of projected max		
Medium-heavy week	indicated % of projected max	−10	−5
Medium week	indicated % of projected max	−20	−10
Light week	indicated % of projected max	−30	−15

For athletes who squat less than 225 pounds and bench press less than 135 pounds

Heavy week	indicated % of projected max		
Medium-heavy week	indicated % of projected max	−5	−5
Medium week	indicated % of projected max	−10	−5
Light week	indicated % of projected max	−15	−10

TABLE 16.2 *Resistance Level for Cycle System*

Monday-Wednesday-Friday

Squat and Bench Press

Weeks	Rating	Weeks	Rating
1) 8-8-5-5-5-5	L	9) 8-8-8-8-8	MH
2) 8-8-5-5-5-5	M	10) 8-8-6-6-5-5	H
3) 8-8-5-5-5-5	MH	11) 8-8-6-6-5-5	L
4) 8-6-4-4-3-3	H	12) 8-8-6-6-5-5	M
5) 8-6-4-4-3-3	MH "Fast"	13) 8-8-5-4-4-4	H
6) 8-6-4-4-3-3	M "Fast"	14) 8-8-5-4-4-4	M
	Indoor Peak		
7) 8-8-8-8-8	L	15) 8-8-5-4-4-4	MH
8) 8-8-8-8-8	M	16) 8-8-5-4-4-4	H

Power Cleans or High Pulls

Weeks	Rating	Weeks	Rating
1) 5-4-4-3-3	L	5) 5-4-3-2-1	MH "Fast"
2) 5-4-4-3-3	M	6) 5-4-3-2-1	M "Fast"
3) 5-4-3-2-2	MH	7) 5-5-5-5	L
4) 5-4-3-2-1	H	8) 5-5-5-5	M

FIGURE 16.14 *Pre-Season Conditioning Program for Shot-Put, Discus, and Javelin (with indoor peak)*

Power Cleans or High Pulls (Continued)

Weeks	Rating	Weeks	Rating
9) 5-5-5-5-5	MH	13) 5-4-3-3-3	H
10) 5-4-3-3-3	H	14) 5-4-3-3-3	M
11) 5-4-4-3-3	L	15) 5-4-3-3-2	MH
12) 5-4-4-3-3	M	16) 5-4-3-3-2	H

"Fast"—Indicates which weeks to increase the speed emphasis.

Supplemental and Specialty Exercises

Bent Arm Laterals***
3 sets, 8 reps

Incline Dumbbell Press**
3 sets, 6 reps

Bent Arm Pullover*
4 sets, 6 reps

Leg Extension
4 sets, 10 reps

Leg Curl
4 sets, 10 reps

Good Morning***, **
Discus: 2 sets, 8 reps
Shot-Put: 2 sets, 6 reps

Hyperextension*
4 sets, 10 reps

Tricep Pushdown
4 sets, 8 reps

Toe Raises
4 sets, 10 reps

Jumping Squats (see Chapter 00, p. 00)
4 sets, 10 reps

Wrist Curls
4 sets, 10 reps

Optional Exercises

Incline Press, Snatch Pull, Military Press.

***Indicates specialty exercises for discus.
**Indicates specialty exercise for shot-put.
*Indicates specialty exercise for javelin.

FIGURE 16.14 *(Continued)*

Monday-Wednesday-Friday

Squat and Bench Press

Weeks	Rating	Weeks	Rating
1) 5-3-3-3-2-2	L	5) 5-3-3-2-2-1	M "Fast"
2) 5-3-3-3-2-2	M "Fast"	6) 5-3-3-2-2-1	H
3) 5-3-3-2-2-2	H	7) 5-3-3-2-2-1	MH "Fast"
4) 5-3-3-3-2-2	L "Fast"	8) 5-3-3-2-2-1	M "Fast"

Power Cleans or High Pulls

Weeks	Rating	Weeks	Rating
1) 5-3-3-2-2-1-1	L	5) 5-3-2-2-1-1-1	M "Fast"
2) 5-3-3-2-2-1-1	M "Fast"	6) 5-3-2-2-1-1-1	H
3) 5-3-3-2-2-1-1	H	7) 5-3-2-2-1-1-1	MH "Fast"
4) 5-3-2-2-1-1-1	L "Fast"	8) 5-3-2-2-1-1-1	M "Fast"

"Fast"—Indicates which weeks to increase speed emphasis.

FIGURE 16.15 *In-Season Conditioning Program for Shot-Put, Discus, and Javelin*

(Continued)

Supplemental and Specialty Exercises

Bent Arm Laterals***
3 sets, 8 reps

Incline Dumbbell Press**
3 sets, 6 reps

Bent Arm Pullover*
3 sets, 6 reps

Leg Extension
4 sets, 8 reps

Leg Curl
4 sets, 8 reps

Good Morning***, **
4 sets, 6 reps

Hyperextension*
4 sets, 10 reps

Triceps Pushdown
4 sets, 6–8 reps

Toe Raises
4 sets, 10 reps

Jumping Squats (p. 00)
4 sets, 8 reps

Wrist Curls
4 sets, 10 reps

***Indicates specialty exercises for discus.
**Indicates specialty exercises for shot-put.
*Indicates specialty exercises for javelin.

FIGURE 16.15 *(Continued)*

for the adjustment sets remember the rule of thumb (Chapter 4, p. 00). "Always make larger or equal increases first."

7. In peaking for important track meets, strict adherence to percentages is waived in favor of a drop in poundages. However, as the emphasis is on speed, the intensity level still remains high as the effective load on the muscles is increased by exploding, or accelerating the resistance.

SUMMARY

Track and field events run the full range of energy mechanisms and skilled activities. Some of the most specific applications of energy mechanisms can be found in track and field events. Stage I anaerobic (ATP-CP) is epitomized by the sprinter at 50 meters, while the marathoner represents the ultimate aerobic (Stage III) athlete. Perhaps no other effort in sport stresses the anaerobic lactic-acid (Stage II) system like a 400-meter run. Strength, explosive power, and flexibility are also epitomized in field events such as shot-putting and high jumping.

Year-round programs for the various track and field events are offered in this chapter. Entire books have been written on a single track event. In the space of this chapter the authors have diligently

attempted to outline the major principles involved in training for track and field events.

REFERENCES

1. Anderson, Bob. "The Perfect Pre-Run Stretching Routine." *Runners' World* (1978) pp. 56–61.
2. Costill, David L. *What Research Tells the Coach about Distance Running.* Washington, D.C.: AAHPER, 1968, 1978.
3. Costill, David L. *A Scientific Approach to Distance Running.* Los Altos, CA: Tafnews Press, 1979.
4. Daniels, Jack; Fitts, Robert; and Sheehan, George. *Conditioning for Distance Running.* New York: John Wiley & Sons, 1978.
5. Dintiman, George B. *What Research Tells the Coach about Sprinting.* Washington, D.C.: AAHPER, 1974.
6. Fox, Edward L., and Matthews, David R. *Interval Training: Conditioning for Sport and Physical Fitness.* Philadelphia: W. B. Saunders Co., 1974.
7. Gowan, G. "Field Events." In *The Scientific Aspects of Sports Training,* A. W. Taylor, ed. Springfield, IL: Charles C. Thomas, 1975, pp. 83–104.
8. Henderson, Joe. "Training to Run Marathons: A Schedule for Runners." *Runners' World* (1978), pp. 74–79.
9. Peronnet, Francois, and Ferguson, Ronald J. "Interval Training." In *The Scientific Aspects of Sports Training,* A. W. Taylor, ed. Springfield, IL: Charles C. Thomas, 1975, pp. 31–41.
10. Wilt, Fred. *The Marathon: Physiological, Medical, Epidemological, and Psychological Studies.* New York: New York Academy of Sciences, 1977.

17

Individual Sports: Archery, Golf, Gymnastics, and Tennis

This chapter contains year-round conditioning programs for archery, golf, gymnastics, and tennis. The programs are designed for the off-season, pre-season, and in-season periods. The reader is referred to four previous chapters for the basis of the programs. In Chapter 3 we discuss aerobic and anaerobic conditioning, in Chapter 4 we describe strength training, in Chapter 5 the authors discuss warm-up, stretching, and flexibility, and in Chapter 8 we outline year-round conditioning. The latter chapter also describes ways of most efficiently putting training objectives together into a single program. The reader is also referred to the sample recording charts offered in the Appendix. These charts will facilitate the measurement of the athlete's progress on the training program and will indicate the athlete's standing in regard to training goals.

ARCHERY

Major conditioning requirements for archery involve *strengthening* the muscles of the upper back, shoulders, and arms, and increasing grip strength. To draw the bow with comparative ease and hold it steady, the archer needs to strengthen the muscles involved. A specific overload exercise for archery would be the repeated drawing of a bow that is heavier than the one used in shooting. Very

few sports offer as specific an example of strength overload as does the use of the heavier bow.

Strength training for archery emphasizes *muscular endurance* as well as muscular strength. Repeated drawing of the bow in a match taxes the local endurance of muscles in the arms and the upper back. Strength training aimed at increasing muscular endurance will involve lighter weight, fast speed, and high-repetition work.[1,2] During the in-season period strength training should be conducted only twice a week, and not before shooting practice. A minor expenditure of time in the in-season program will maintain strength for the archer. Flexibility exercises can be practiced by the archer on a year-round or a maintenance schedule.

Off-season, pre-season, and in-season conditioning programs for archery are offered in Figures 17.1, 17.2, and 17.3.

REFERENCES

1. Dannock, Joanne. "Archery: From the Backwoods to the Weight Room." *Scholastic Coach* (1977), pp. 64–65.
2. Stone, William J. "Some Scientific Aspects of Archery." In *Target Archery*, M. L. Klann. Reading, MA: Addison-Wesley Publishing Co. 1970, pp. 105–111.

Warm-Up and Stretching

Strength Training—Train Explosively!

Monday & Friday
Bench Press
5–8 sets, 10-10-8-6-4-2

Half-Squat or Leg Extension
5–8 sets, 8-8-6-6-4-4

Bent Over Rowing (with dumbbells;
hold flexed position 1–5 secs.)
5 sets, 8–15 reps

Wrist Roller and/or Wrist Curl
3–5 sets

Archery Bow Drawing Motion (with pulley)
5 sets, 10 reps

Sit-Ups and/or Leg Lifts
5 sets, 10–25 reps

Good Morning or Hyperextension
5 sets, 10 reps

Upright Rowing
5 sets, 6–10 reps

*Lateral Raises
5 sets, 10–15 reps

*Side Bends (with dumbbells)
5 sets, 10–15 reps

Cable Curls
5 sets, 10–15 reps

Optional Exercises
Toe Raises, Arm Circles, Bent Arm Pullover.

Stretching Exercises

*Light weight, fast speed, high reps

Wednesday
Military or Incline Press
5–8 sets, 10-10-8-6-4-2

Half-Squat or Leg Extension
5–8 sets, 8-8-6-6-4-4

Wrist Roller and/or Wrist Curl
3–5 sets

Archery Bow Drawing Motion
(with pulley)
5 sets, 10 reps

Sit-Ups and/or Leg Lifts
5 sets, 10–25 reps

Good Morning or Hyperextension
5 sets, 10 reps

Upright Rowing
5 sets, 6–10 reps

*Lateral Raises
5 sets, 10–15 reps

*Side Bends (with dumbbells)
5 sets, 10–15 reps

FIGURE 17.1   *Off-Season Conditioning Program for Archery*

Warm-Up and Stretching

Strength Training—Train Explosively!

Monday & Friday
Bench Press
3–8 sets, 10-10-8-6-4-2

Half-Squat or Leg Extension
3–8 sets, 8-8-8-8-6-6

Bent Over Rowing (with dumbbells;
hold flexed position 1–5 secs.)
3–5 sets, 10–20 reps

Wednesday
Military or Incline Press
3–8 sets, 10-10-8-6-4-2

Half-Squat or Leg Extension
3–8 sets, 8-8-8-8-6-6

Bent Over Rowing (with dumbbells;
hold flexed position 1–5 secs.)
3–5 sets, 10–20 reps

FIGURE 17.2   *Pre-Season Conditioning Program for Archery*

(Continued)

Monday & Friday

Wrist Roller and/or Wrist Curl
3–5 sets

Archery Bow Drawing Motion
3–5 sets, 10–20 reps

Sit-Ups and/or Leg Lifts
3–5 sets, 10–50 reps

Good Morning or Hyperextension
3–5 sets, 10–20 reps

Upright Rowing
3–5 sets, 10–15 reps

*Lateral Raises
3–5 sets, 10–25 reps

*Side Bends (with dumbbells)
3–5 sets, 10–25 reps

Cable Curls
3–5 sets, 10–15 reps

Optional Exercises
Toe Raises, Arm Circles, Bent Arm Pullover.

Stretching Exercises

 *Light weight, fast speed, high reps

Wednesday

Wrist Roller and/or Wrist Curl
3–5 sets

Archery Bow Drawing Motion
3–5 sets, 10–20 reps

Sit-Ups and/or Leg Lifts
3–5 sets, 10–50 reps

Good Morning or Hyperextension
3–5 sets, 10–20 reps

Upright Rowing
3–5 sets, 10–15 reps

*Lateral Raises
3–5 sets, 10–25 reps

*Side Bends (with dumbbells)
3–5 sets, 10–25 reps

FIGURE 17.2 *(Continued)*

Warm-Up and Stretching

Strength Training—Train Explosively!

Monday & Wednesday

Bench Press
2–5 sets, 10-10-8-8-6-6

Bent Over Rowing (with dumbbells)
and/or Archery Bow Drawing Motion
2–3 sets, 10–20 reps

Wrist Roller and/or Wrist Curl
2–3 sets

*Side Bends
2–3 sets, 10–25 reps

Optional Exercises
Toe Raises, Sit-Ups, Leg Lifts, Good Morning, Hyperextension, Upright Rowing, Lateral Raises, Arm Circles, Bent Arm Pullover, Cable Curls.

Stretching Exercises

 *Light weight, fast speed, high reps

FIGURE 17.3 *In-Season Conditioning Program for Archery*

GOLF

The golf swing is strictly an *anaerobic* action. The primary conditioning would involve strengthening of the grip, arms, shoulders, and back. Since the game is played for a period of several hours and includes walking over sometimes hilly terrain, *aerobic* capacity is also involved in playing the game of golf. Tournaments are played over several consecutive days, and the cumulative effect challenges the local muscular endurance in the legs.

Strength training for golf is aimed primarily at the upper body, particularly the shoulders, arms, and forearms, and grip strength. The legs are also involved in developing power in the swing. The emphasis is on lighter resistance, many repetitions, and high-speed strength training. Training of that nature develops muscular endurance as well as strength. A two-day-a-week in-season program will help a golfer maintain muscular strength and aerobic condition with a minimum expenditure of time.

Another important facet of the golf game is flexibility. The number of strokes both in practice and in tournament conditions place significant stress on the golfer's musculoskeletal system, especially the back. A year-round stretching program should be developed and maintained.

Off-season, pre-season, and in-season condi-

tioning programs for golf are listed in Figures 17.4, 17.5, and 17.6.

GYMNASTICS

The major conditioning requirements for gymnastics involves *upper body strength:* shoulders, abdominals, arms, and grip strength. Many events also require a great amount of explosive leg power. The practice of gymnastics routines produces some strength training. Gymnasts must maintain strength and performance condition practically year round, hence a year round conditioning program is almost essential.

Until recently, most gymnasts used the resistance involved in their routines to develop specific strength. Boone,[1] however, has noted that most gymnastics skills require strength for proper execution, and that strength should be developed first, before muscular endurance. He suggests a

---

Warm-Up and Stretching

Aerobic Conditioning

		Distance	*% Max.*	*Time (approx.)*
Run:		2–3 mi.	75%	14–24:00 mins.

Strength Training—Train Explosively!

Monday & Friday
Bench Press
5–10 sets (A) 10-10-8-8-8-8-6-6
           (B) 20-20-8-8-6-6-4-4
Half-Squat
5–8 sets (A) 8-8-8-8-6-6-6-6
        (B) 8-8-8-6-6-6-4-4
Reverse Curl
5 sets, 10 reps
Side Bends
5 sets, 10 reps
Wrist Roller and/or Wrist Curls
3–5 sets
Wrist Extension
3–5 sets, 10–25 reps
Golf Swing
5 sets, 10 reps
Sit-Ups
5 sets, 10–50 reps

Stretching Exercises

Wednesday
Incline or Military Press
5–8 sets, 10-8-8-6-6
Lat Pulls
5 sets, 10 reps
Jumping Squats
5 sets, 10–15 reps
Reverse Curl
5 sets, 10 reps
Side Bends
5 sets, 10 reps
Wrist Roller and/or Wrist Curls
3–5 sets
Wrist Extension
3–5 sets, 10–25 reps
Golf Swing
5 sets, 10 reps
Sit-Ups
5 sets, 10–50 reps

FIGURE 17.4 *Off-Season Conditioning Program for Golf*

Warm-Up and Stretching

Aerobic Conditioning

	Distance	% Max.	Time (approx.)
Run:	2–3 mi.	85%	14–22:00 mins.

Strength Training—Train Explosively!

Monday-Wednesday-Friday

Bench Press
3–5 sets, 6–10 reps

Incline or Military Press
2–5 sets, 6–10 reps

Half-Squat or Jumping Squat
3–5 sets, 6–10 reps

Golf Swing (with pulley)
2–5 sets, 10–15 reps

Reverse Curl
2–5 sets, 10 reps

Wrist Extension
2–5 sets, 10–25 reps

Side Bends
2–5 sets, 10–15 reps

Lat Pull or Bent Over Rowing
2–5 sets, 10 reps

Wrist Roller and/or Wrist Curls
2–5 sets

Sit-Ups
2–5 sets, 10–50 reps

Stretching Exercises

FIGURE 17.5 *Pre-Season Conditioning Program for Golf*

Warm-Up and Stretching

Aerobic Conditioning

	Distance	% Max.	Time (approx.)
Run:	2–3 mi.	95%	14–22:00 mins.

Strength Training—Train Explosively!

Monday & Wednesday

Wrist Roller and/or Wrist Curl
2–3 sets

Golf Swing (with pulley)
2–3 sets, 10–15 reps

Side Bends
2–3 sets, 10–15 reps

Sit-Ups
2–5 sets, 10–50 reps

Optional Exercises

Half-Squat, Leg Extension, Bench Press, Reverse Curl, Incline Press, Military Press, Bar Dips, Wrist Extension, Bent Arm Pullover, Lat Pull, Bent Over Rowing.

Stretching Exercises

FIGURE 17.6 *In-Season Conditioning Program for Golf*

combination of progressive resistance (weights or machines) and resistance while practicing gymnastics skills. It is important to remember that resistance to the skill before it can be executed properly violates the principle of motor skill specificity. Allen has also acknowledged the need to use weight training or weight machines to develop sufficient strength.[2] He also utilizes resistance while practicing specific routines through the use of a partner.

Some specific gymnastics routines (such as vaulting) require running speed and leg power. *Anaerobic* sprints should be used to condition the gymnast for such events. Sprints in the range of twenty-five to fifty yards are required to develop anaerobic leg power (speed and acceleration).

During the off-season the gymnast may concentrate on developing greater amounts of strength, thus the time spent in the conditioning program should be proportionately greater than that spent in skills practice. While the intensity may increase, the time spent on strength training during the pre-season period will diminish. During the in-season period a minimum of time (one to two sessions per week) will be sufficient to maintain strength. At any time during the year-round regimen the gymnast may desire to use strength training designed specifically for one event. The necessary strength to perform some gymnastic routines may not be developed until a specific strength training program is devised and followed.

Off-season, pre-season, and in-season conditioning programs for gymnastics are offered in Figures 17.7, 17.8, and 17.9.

Warm-Up and Stretching

Strength Training—Train Explosively!

Monday & Friday

Military or Incline Press
6–12 sets, 10-10-8-6-4-2-1-1-4-4-6-6

Bench Press (with dumbbells)
3–5 sets, 6–10 reps

Half-Squat
6–10 sets, 8-8-8-6-4-2-2-2

Toe Raises
5–8 sets, 30 reps

Lat Pulls or Bent Over Rowing
5 sets, 10-10-8-8-8

Wrist Roller and/or Wrist Curls
3–5 sets

Sit-Ups and/or Leg Lifts (upright position, with ankle weights)
3–5 sets, 10–50 reps

*Stiff-legged Dead Lift, Hyperextension, and/or Good Morning
3–5 sets, 10–15 reps

Upright Rowing
3–5 sets, 8–10 reps

Straight Arm Pulldown (with pulley, using handgrips or bar)
3–5 sets, 8–15 reps

Ankle Exercises
5 sets

Wednesday

Bench Press
6–12 sets, 10-10-8-6-4-4-4-4-4

Bar Dips
6–8 sets, 10-10-8-8-8-8-6-6

Jumping Squat
5–8 sets, 10-10-8-8-8-8

Toe Raises
5–8 sets, 30 reps

Lat Pulls or Bent Over Rowing
5 sets, 10-10-8-8-8

Wrist Roller and/or Wrist Curls
3–5 sets

Specialty Exercises

Movements with resistance and range of motion imitative of the power phase of the particular gymnastic trick.

Still Rings
  A. Iron Cross movement (with pulleys)
  B. Lateral Raises
  C. Straight Arm Pulldown (with handgrips or rings on pulleys)

Horizontal Bar and Uneven Bar
  Straight Arm Pulldown (i.e., Kip movement, with bar on pulley)

Parallel Bars
  Bar Dips (2–3 days per week)

FIGURE 17.7 *Off-Season Conditioning Program for Gymnastics*

Specialty Exercises (Continued)

Floor Exercise and Tumbling, Vaulting
  A. Jumping Squats (2–3 days per week)
  B. Hyperextension (2–3 days per week)

Side Horse
  Lateral Leg Lifts (with ankle weights or pulley)

Balance Beam
  Good Morning
  Ankle Exercises

Optional Exercises
  Lateral Raises, Bent Arm Pullover, Triceps Extension, Leg Extension, Clean.

Stretching Exercises

  *Light weight, fast speed, high reps

FIGURE 17.7 *(Continued)*

Warm-Up and Stretching

Strength Exercises—Train Explosively!

Monday & Friday

Military or Incline Press
3–8 sets, 6–10 reps

Bench Press (with dumbbells)
3–5 sets, 6–10 reps

Jumping Squat
3–5 sets, 8–15 reps

Toe Raises
3–8 sets, 30 reps

Lat Pulls or Bent Over Rowing
3–5 sets, 8–15 reps

Wrist Roller and/or Wrist Curls
3–5 sets

Sit-Ups and/or Leg Lifts (upright position, with ankle weights)
3–5 sets, 10–50 reps

Stiff-legged Dead Lift, Hyperextension, and/or Good Morning
3–5 sets, 10–20 reps

Upright Rowing
3–5 sets, 8–12 reps

Straight Arm Pulldown (with pulley)
3–5 sets, 10–15 reps

Ankle Exercises
3–5 sets

Wednesday

Bench Press
3–8 sets, 6–10 reps

Bar Dips
3–8 sets, 6–10 reps

Jumping Squat
3–5 sets, 8–15 reps

Toe Raises
3–8 sets, 30 reps

Specialty Exercises

Movements with resistance and range of motion imitative of the power phase of the particular gymnastic trick.

Still Rings
  A. Iron Cross movement (with pulleys)
  B. Lateral Raises
  C. Straight Arm Pulldown (with handgrips or rings on pulleys)

FIGURE 17.8 *Pre-Season Conditioning Program for Gymnastics*

Specialty Exercises

Horizontal Bar and Uneven Bar
   Straight Arm Pulldown (i.e., Kip movement, with bar on pulley)

Parallel Bars
   Bar Dips (2–3 days per week)

Floor Exercise and Tumbling, Vaulting
   A. Jumping Squats (2–3 days per week)
   B. Hyperextension (2–3 days per week)

Side Horse
   Lateral Leg Lifts (with ankle weights or pulley)

Balance Beam
   Good Morning
   Ankle Exercises

Optional Exercises

Lateral Raises, Bent Arm Pullover, Triceps Extension, Leg Extension, Clean.

Stretching Exercises

FIGURE 17.8 *(Continued)*

Warm-Up and Stretching

Strength Training—Train Explosively!

Monday & Wednesday

Military or Incline Press	Lat Pulls or Bent Over Rowing
2–3 sets, 8–10 reps	2–3 sets, 8–12 reps
Jumping Squat	Ankle Exercise
2–3 sets, 8–20 reps	2–3 sets
Wrist Roller and/or Wrist Curl	
2–3 sets	

Specialty Exercises

Movements with resistance and range of motion imitative of the power phase of the particular gymnastic trick.

Still Rings
   A. Iron Cross movement (with pulleys)
   B. Lateral Raises
   C. Straight Arm Pulldown (with handgrips or rings on pulleys)

Horizontal Bar and Uneven Bar
   Straight Arm Pulldown (i.e., Kip movement, with bar on pulley)

Parallel Bars
   Bar Dips (2–3 days per week)

Floor Exercise and Tumbling, Vaulting
   A. Jumping Squats
   B. Hyperextension (2–3 days per week)

Side Horse
   Lateral Leg Lifts (with ankle weights or pulley)

FIGURE 17.9 *In-Season Conditioning Program for Gymnastics*

Specialty Exercises (Continued)

Balance Beam
  Good Morning
  Ankle Exercise

Optional Exercises
Toe Raises, Sit-Ups, Leg Lifts (with ankle weights), Stiff-legged Dead Lift, Hyperextension, Good Morning, Upright Rowing.

Stretching Exercises

FIGURE 17.9 *(Continued)*

SUMMARY

The primary requirements for gymnasts are upper body strength and explosive leg power. Gymnastics is a very anaerobic sport, and only during free exercise routines does the gymnast wander out of the anaerobic Stage I (ATP-CP). Flexibility is a major component also of gymnastics and should be maintained year round. Year round programs aimed at improving the components of gymnastics are included in this chapter.

REFERENCES

1. Boone, Tommy. "Muscle Strength and Gymnastics." In *Toward an Understanding of Human Performance,* Edmund J. Burke, ed. 2d ed. Ithaca, NY: Mouvement Publications, 1980.
2. Goranson, Gary. "Kip Strength: Explosive Power for Olympic Gymnasts." *NSCA Journal* 3 (1981): 4-6, 55.

TENNIS

Even the shortest tennis match will likely involve at least an hour of continuous movement and play. Matches can last much longer, and the major contributing factor to this requirement is *aerobic* power. Quick and explosive movements are also characteristic of tennis, and they involve *anaerobic* leg power. Local muscular endurance in both the legs and arms is also challenged by tennis. Properly played, tennis can be a very vigorous game requiring a high level of physical conditioning.

Tennis can also be played in short anaerobic bursts averaging two to three seconds, with ten to fifteen seconds between serves. In that respect it resembles football, although there is a longer rest period between football plays. Stewart[3] has identified aerobic power, anaerobic leg power, strength, and agility as the major factors in play. Although extraordinarily short matches have been known to last only fifteen to twenty minutes, most last over an hour, and the extremely lengthy matches can drag on for hours. The longer, hard-fought matches are a real test of endurance for the athlete. The repetitious use and force involved in hitting the ball results in the classic hypertrophy and strength increase in the dominant arm.[2] The need for *agility* and *flexibility* is also high in tennis, and a well-planned stretching program should be conducted year round.[1]

During the off-season a great deal of emphasis can be directed toward the development of aerobic leg power and muscular strength. In the pre-season period the aerobic conditioning becomes more intense through the use of aerobic intervals. They are designed to bring the tennis player to peak condition in a brief period of time. During the in-season period aerobic condition can be maintained, as can strength, with a two-day-a-week program. Strength training should emphasize fast-speed, low-resistance, high-repetition work designed to increase muscular endurance in the arms and legs. Local muscular endurance is an essential part of tennis, as the player may take hundreds of strokes in a single match. Each stroke requires that the player get into a good hitting position, make the stroke, and return to the READY position. Repeating this sequence hundreds of times can be done effectively only if the tennis player is well-conditioned.

During the season the coach or athlete can use the practice time for aerobic or anaerobic conditioning. Continuous play without interruption will aid in the development of aerobic power. Drills requiring quick action and acceleration, repeated over and over, will aid in the development of anaerobic power. Skill drills help to develop local muscular endurance for specific strokes.

Off-season, pre-season, and in-season conditioning programs for tennis are offered in Figures 17.10, 17.11, and 17.12.

SPECIALTY EXERCISES

Bow Drawing Motion (with wall pulley)

This exercise is done with a wall pulley at shoulder height. The exact motion used to draw the bow should be followed, with the bow arm extended against the wall or a stationary object. See Photo 17.1.

Warm-Up and Stretching

Aerobic Conditioning

	Distance	% Max.	Time (approx.)
Run:	2–3 mi.	75–85%	14–24:00 mins.

Strength Training—Train Explosively!

Monday & Friday	Wednesday
Bench Press 6 sets, 10-10-8-8-8-8	Incline Press 6 sets, 10-10-8-8-8-8
Throwing Pullover 5 sets, 10 reps	Upright Rowing 5 sets, 10 reps
Half-Squat 6 sets, 10-10-8-8-8-8	Good Mornings 5 sets, 10 reps
Toe Raises 6 sets, 30 reps	Toe Raises 6 sets, 30 reps
Forehand Motion (with wall pulley) 5 sets, 10 reps	Forehand Motion (with wall pulley) 5 sets, 10 reps
Backhand Motion 5 sets, 10 reps	Backhand Motion 5 sets, 10 reps
Sit-Ups (twisting) 5 sets, 10–25 reps	Sit-Ups (twisting) 5 sets, 10–25 reps
Wrist Curl 3–5 sets	Wrist Curl 3–5 sets
Arm Circles 3–5 sets, 10–50 reps	Arm Circles 3–5 sets, 10–50 reps

Optional Exercises

Lateral Raises, Incline Flys, Leg Extension, Leg Curl (toes in), Throwing Pullover, Ankle Exercise.

Stretching Exercises

FIGURE 17.10 *Off-Season Conditioning Program for Tennis*

Warm-Up and Stretching

Aerobic Conditioning

	Distance	% Max.	Rest	Reps
Run:	880 yds.	95%↑	3 mins.	4–6

Strength Training—Train Explosively!

FIGURE 17.11 *Pre-Season Conditioning Program for Tennis*

(Continued)

Monday-Wednesday-Friday

Bench Press (with dumbbells, optional) 3–6 sets, 10–15 reps	Jumping Squat (or Fast Speed Machine) 3–6 sets, 10–15 reps
Serving Motion (with wall pulley) 3–5 sets, 10–15 reps	Sit-Ups (twisting) 3–6 sets, 10–50 reps
Forehand Motion (with wall pulley) 3–5 sets, 10–15 reps	Toe Raises 3–6 sets, 30 reps
Backhand Motion (with wall pulley) 3–5 sets, 10–15 reps	Arm Circles 3–5 sets, 10–20 reps
Wrist Curl 3–5 sets	

Optional Exercises

Lateral Raises, Incline Flys, Leg Extension, Leg Curl (toes in), Throwing Pullover, Ankle Exercise.

Stretching Exercises

FIGURE 17.11 *(Continued)*

Warm-Up and Stretching

Aerobic Conditioning

	Distance	% Max.	Time (approx.)
Run:	2–3 mi.	95%↑	14–22:00 mins.

Strength Training—Train Explosively!

Monday & Wednesday

Bench Press (with dumbbells, optional) 2–3 sets, 8–15 reps	Wrist Curl 2–3 sets
Serving Motion (with wall pulley) 2–3 sets, 10–15 reps	Jumping Squat 2–3 sets, 10–15 reps
Forehand Motion (with wall pulley) 2–3 sets, 10–15 reps	Sit-Ups 2–3 sets, 10–50 reps
Backhand Motion (with wall pulley) 2–3 sets, 10–15 reps	Toe Raises 2–3 sets, 30–75 reps

Optional Exercises

Arm Circles, Lateral Raises, Incline Flys, Leg Extension, Leg and Curl (toes in), Throwing Pullover, Ankle Exercise.

Stretching Exercises

FIGURE 17.12 *In-Season Conditioning Program for Tennis*

Golf Swing

This exercise employs a high pulley attached to a wall pulley to imitate the range of motion against resistance.

Straight Arm Pulldown (with hand grips, bar, and rings)

This exercise imitates the Kip movement. In the standing position using a high pulley or pulleys,

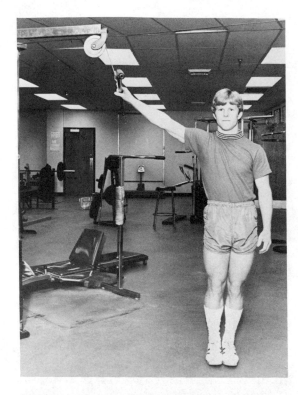

with the arms completely extended, pull the resistance down directly in front of the body.

Iron Cross

This exercise is similar to the Straight Arm Pulldown, using high pulleys to pull downward, with extended arms. In the Iron Cross, of course, the arms are extended to the side instead of in front.

Dorsiflexion of the Foot

(See Chapter 6.)

REFERENCES

1. Anderson, Bob. "For Tennis: Stretching Works When Done Correctly." *NSCA Journal* 3 (1981): 18–20.
2. Grey, Mervin R. *What Research Tells the Coach about Tennis.* Washington, D.C.: AAHPER, 1974.
3. Stewart, Kerry J. "Conditioning for Tennis: Some Basic Considerations." In *Toward an Understanding of Human Performance*, Edmund J. Burke, ed. 2d ed. Ithaca, NY: Mouvement Publications, 1980.

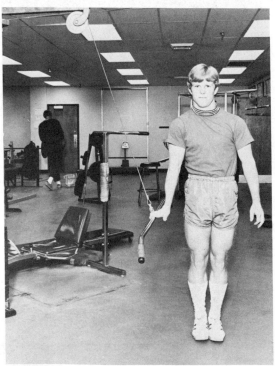

PHOTO 17.1　*Iron Cross*

Appendix

TESTS OF AEROBIC POWER

1.0 Introduction

There are several running tests to use in estimating aerobic power. Two standard tests are: a) the 12-Minute Run for distance and b) the 1.5 Mile Run for time. Either of these tests can be administered easily with an entire team in less than thirty minutes. They each require only a track and a stopwatch, but the 1.5-Mile Run is easier to score and maintain records of progress.

2.0 Procedures

A. Each player selects a partner. One-half of the the team takes the test at one time while the other half records distance (12-Minute Run) *or* time (1.5-Mile Run).
B. The coach "starts" the run and athletes continue for 12 minutes or 1.5 miles, depending upon the test selected.
C. The object of the test is to run as far as possible in 12 minutes or to run 1.5 miles as fast as possible.
D. At the conclusion of the test, the partner

Score	Males	Test	Females
Excellent	1.73 Mi.↑	12-Min. Run	1.27 Mi.↑
	9.:40 Mins.↓	1.5-Mi. Run	14:00 Mins.↓
Good	1.60–1.72	12-Min. Run	1.16–1.26
	9:41–10:35	1.5-Mi. Run	14:01–15:25
Fair	1.47–1.59	12-Min. Run	1.06–1.16
	10:36–11:30	1.5-Mi. Run	17:00–15:25

APPENDIX 2.1 *Aerobic Power Scores: Junior High School and High School (13–18 Yrs.)*

Score	Males	Test	Females
Excellent	2.0 Mi.↑	12-Min. Run	1.65 Mi.↑
	9:00 Mins.↓	1.5-Mi. Run	11:00 Mins.↓
Good	1.75–2.0	12-Min. Run	1.35–1.64
	9:01–10:29	1.5-Mi. Run	11:00–11:59
Fair	1.50–1.75	12-Min. Run	1.15–1.34
	10:30–12:00	1.5-Mi. Run	12:00–15:59

APPENDIX 2.2 *Aerobic Power Scores: College Age and Above (19–29 Yrs.)*

records the distance *or* time and the athletes trade places.

3.0 Scoring

Note: The attached scoring tables for aerobic power are only suggested. Your athletes, because of sport or age, may have noticeably greater or less aerobic power. The scoring table should serve as a guideline, and with repeated testing of your athletes you can develop your own scale for aerobic power.

TEST OF ANAEROBIC POWER

1.0 Introduction

Anaerobic power is extremely important in athletics, since many athletic skills are quick and explosive, lasting only a few seconds. A simple test of anaerobic power was devised by Margaria, and requires only a solid flight of stairs and a stopwatch readable to .01 seconds.

2.0 Procedures

A. Use stairs (12-16) with a 6–8" rise, and weigh the subject before the test.
B. Position the subject six feet in front of the first step and require a *maximal effort* from the start to beyond the twelfth step.
C. The subject takes *two steps at a time*, and the

stopwatch is started as the foot hits the *fourth step*. The stopwatch is stopped as the same foot hits the *twelfth step*. (The subject is assumed to have reached peak acceleration at the fourth step.)

D. Allow the subject *three* trials, with two to three minutes rest between trials. Record each trial and average the three.

3.0 Recording

See recording form.

EQUIPMENT

There are many pieces of equipment that accompany free weights, such as: bench with racks for Bench Press; rack for Squats and Military Press; power rack; calf machine; neck harness; straps for High Pulls and Dead Lifts; and the weight belt. All equipment should be kept sturdy and safe with proper padding and a minimum of sharp corners or edges.

Bench

The bench should be about fifteen to eighteen inches high and from ten to twelve inches wide, with approximately an inch of padding. The rack for an Olympic bar should be wider than that for the standard bar. The rack should allow the bar to rest approximately three feet from the floor, in easy position to be removed for bench pressing.

Wt. (lbs.) ___200___ Vertical rise: 8 steps X (6") = ___4___ feet.

Test trials 1. _____ 2. _____ 3. _____ (T) AVG. ___2___ .8 1.6

Work (ft.-lbs.) = F X D
   W = Wt. (200) X Vertical Rise (4)
   W = ___800___ ft.-lbs.   200 .73
                                               180 .65
Power (Work per unit time) = W (800)   220 .80
               Time Avg. (2) = ft.-lbs./sec.

Power (hp) = P ( )
      550 ft.-lbs./sec. = ___2.9___ hp.   3.2 3.6

Vertical speed = $\frac{D}{T}$ = _____ = _____ ft./sec.

Anaerobic Power Trial Record

(Mon.)	Dist.	Time	HR-	(Wed.)	Dist.	Time	HR	(Fri.)	Dist.	Time	HR	Wk.

Name _____   Max. HR _____

Aerobic-Anaerobic Performance Chart

Date	Exercise & No. of Sets													
	Wt.													
	Reps.													

Strength Recording Sheet

If more than one bench is used, it would be advisable to vary the size slightly to accommodate athletes of various sizes.

Squat Rack

The squat rack for Squats and Military Presses should be adjustable, if possible; if not, the preferred height is about two inches to four inches below shoulder level.

Power Rack

The power rack can be used for a variety of exercises. The Military Press, Rack Squat, Rack Bench, and Rack Dead Lift are the most common. The exercise is done with the bar inside the rack. The pins in the rack can be adjusted so that the bar can be elevated to any level. By using two sets of pins, isometric exercises or partial isometric contractions requiring a minimum level of intensity can be done on the power rack.

Calf Machine

Various types of calf machines are available. The standard hinge type is sufficient. Many other types of equipment can be used for toe raises. The power rack, for instance, is adaptable to this exercise.

Neck Harness

The neck harness is a simple item that can vary greatly in quality. It is most important that the neck harness be comfortable, strong, and durable.

Pull Straps

These are usually about one inch wide and two feet long. They must be made of a tough cotton and/or nylon interwoven material.

Weight Belt

The weight belt is used to give needed support to the back and abdomen. The official competition weight-lifting belt can be no more than four inches wide at any point. In some cases athletes might wish to use a slightly wider belt since weight training is noncompetitive.

Cybex II

The Cybex II (Lumex, Inc.) is a sophisticated isokinetic device that can be used by athletes for strength development and the prevention and rehabilitation of injuries. The machine can be used to exercise the hips, knees, ankles, wrists, elbows, or shoulders. An electromagnetic device controls the speed of the isokinetic movements very accurately. The speed ranges vary from isometric to those well above human capabilities. The potentials of this machine are enhanced by the strip chart recording capabilities. The fact that both flexion and extension are exercised in a single repetition is advantageous, and the possibility of preventing injuries by systematic testing and early diagnosis of personal physical weaknesses exists.

Orthotron and Cybex Power Press

The *Orthotron* and Cybex Power Press Systems (Lumex, Inc.) have the identical isokinetic characteristics and capabilities as the Cybex II, but the testing and recording capabilities of the Cybex are not included. The Cybex Power Press Systems utilize the Leg Press and Bench Press movements.

Marcy's Circuit Trainer

Marcy's Circuit Trainer includes sixteen different exercise stations. Exercises include Bench Press, Leg Drive, Chinning, isometric power rack, Military Press, Lat machine, high and low pulleys, Sit-up board, Hyperextension station, Leg Extension (or quad and ham) machine, Hip Flexion station, Wrist Roller, Neck Extension, and Dip station.

Mini Gym

The Mini Gym 101 is a variable speed isokinetic device. It can be used alternatively as a wall pulley for specialized movements or from the floor for Deadlift Clean, Military Press, Bent Over Row, or Curl. The Model 180 includes a gauge with two hands, indicating present and maximum force. A number of accessories can be attached to the

Mini Gym 101

Mini Gym 101 or other Mini Gym equipment to provide a variety of specialty exercises. Included in this category are isokinetic machines used to appropriate major power exercises such as the Military Press and Deadlift.

Mini Gym Isokinetic Power Rack. This device is capable of many movements: High Pulls (close or wide grip), Squats, Deadlifts, Military Press, Bench Press, Triceps Extension, Toe Raises, Close Grip Bench Press, and Bent Over Row. Variable isokinetic resistance can be produced.

Mini Gym Isokinetic Squat Thrust. The Squat Thrust is excellent for developing leg, hip, and back strength for athletes.

Mini Gym Isokinetic Bench Press. The Bench Press is a major strength developing movement for the upper body of the athlete.

Mini Gym Isokinetic Quadriceps and Hamstrings. This machine is effective in the rehabilitation and prevention of knee injuries as well as general thigh development.

Some machines used for specialized purposes include:

Mini Gym Squat Thrust

Mini Gym Bench Press

Mini Gym Swim Bench

Mini Gym Swim Bench

- Isokinetic Super Runner
- Leaper
- Leaper for Women
- Isokinetic Swim Bench
- Isokinetic Baseball Machine
- Isokinetic Rehabilitation Unit
- Isokinetic Gymnastic Strength Unit
- Women's Isokinetic Stations
- Four-Station Circuit for Swimmers
- Gymnastics Circuit

Nautilus (Sports/Medical Industries)

The Nautilus equipment is effective in developing strength for athletes year round and for the prevention and rehabilitation of injuries and the improvement of athletic performance. The manufacturer recommends a specific type of strength training to be used with this equipment. Because of the nature of the Nautilus equipment, the recommended programs should be followed. Resis-

tance will change throughout the full range of motion.

The Universal Gym (Universal Athletic Sales)

The Universal Gym is an effective machine in developing strength for athletes year round. The *Universal Centurion* can be obtained in units of up to sixteen stations. All of the major strength exercises are included. They are the Leg Press, Bench Press (Chest Press), Military Press (Shoulder Press), Chinning Station, High Lat Pull station, Quad and Dead Lift station, Dipping station, Hip Flexor, Abdominal Conditioner (Sit-up board), Thigh-knee machine, Back hyper-station and Swimmer's Kick station, Rowing station, Wrist Conditioner, Neck Conditioner, Hand Gripper Station, and Real Runner.

A feature of the Universal Gym called Variable Resistance allows the amount of resistance to be varied to accommodate the athlete's capability at every point in the range of motion. The Universal Centurion is a model containing eleven stations.

Universal Centurion

Single stations with the Variable Resistance are the Chest Press (Bench Press), Leg Press, and Shoulder Press.

Free Weights

There are two types of free weights, Olympic weights and standard one-inch barbells—also various types of dumbbells and fixed-weight barbells. Many companies manufacture weights in essentially the same form, thus the plates and bars of different brands are generally interchangeable.